"I will definitely re-read Noah Karrasch
use it as a text for yoga teacher and yoga therapy ...
work integrates all of the top thinkers on fascia, vagus, mind/body,
energy, and healing into a readable and useful model that helps
therapists remember why we do this healing work."
—*Beth Spindler C-IAYT, ERYT500, Yoga Therapist,*
Teacher, and Writer at Yoga International Publications

"Noah's book is a profound integration of cutting-edge concepts in
physiology, health, and integrative medicine. In my view, this book
(especially the first five chapters) should be required reading for all
healers, beginning with physicians of all specialities, psychologists,
and therapists of any persuasion. His understanding of the autonomic
nervous system, and the impact of heart rate variability on overall
health and function, is a must-read for any health practitioner. He
makes very difficult material easy to understand.

The second half of the book will be of great value to any
bodyworker/movement therapist. Noah's practical applications of
his bodymindcore concepts are useful, and helpful.

As a client/patient, I have frequently benefited from Noah's
bodymindcore work. He helps me breathe, move, and grow in a
way that few others can."
—*Ralph Harvey, MD, Cornerstone*
Family Practice, MI, USA

"This easy-to-read book thoughtfully shares Noah's wisdoms gleaned
from a lifetime of living with the process of healing the bodymind.
He adds to the deepness of his extensive experience by grounding
it within the research and practice of other contemporary leaders
in the field. I plan to keep this resource handy to read whenever my
physical listening senses need a honing!"
—*Victoria Day, MEd, PLPC, certification student LIMS*

"I have had over 50 sessions with Noah and consider his work
at the top of the bodywork movement. Read and heed this
inspirational message."
—*C. Norman Shealy, MD, PhD, Founder and CEO,*
International Institute of Holistic Medicine

"Weaving insights from body-centered therapeutic realms, mind-centered psychology, and heart-centered practices such as yoga, Noah Karrasch has created a wonderful synergy between Western practicalities and Eastern modalities. Yoga teachers, of which I am one, will benefit from hearing what he has to say, as will their students."

—Bernie Clark, author of Your Body, Your Yoga, and
The Complete Guide to Yin Yoga

"Having worked in the fitness and bodywork industry for over two decades, I've had the privilege to be taught by the inspirational and knowledgeable Noah Karrasch. His unique approach combines decades of study, knowledge, and personal experience. I have passed on his hidden gems and techniques to hundreds of my own students over the years with startling and profound results. His model, philosophy, and approach give guaranteed results.

Noah shares his perspective on opening and loosening the bodymindcore, in order to unwind and release inner tension. This tension can cause a reduction in circulation, resulting in a lack of energy within the body, often leading to pain.

Whether you are a bodywork professional or enthusiast, there is something for everybody in this book, due to Noah's clear and concise explanation. A fascinating read—highly recommended!"

—Emma Newham, Director, Pilates Union UK, Creator of the
BarreConcept Method, and Owner of MyBody Studios

BodyMindCORE Work

FOR THE MOVEMENT THERAPIST

by the same author

Meet Your Body
CORE Bodywork and Rolfing Tools to Release Bodymindcore Trauma
Noah Karrasch
Illustrated by Lovella Lindsey Norrell
ISBN 978 1 84819 016 0
eISBN 978 0 85701 000 1

Freeing Emotions and Energy Through Myofascial Release
Noah Karrasch
ISBN 978 1 84819 085 6
eISBN 978 0 85701 065 0

Getting Better at Getting People Better
Creating Successful Therapeutic Relationships
Noah Karrasch
ISBN 978 1 84819 239 3
eISBN 978 0 85701 186 2

BodyMindCORE Work

FOR THE MOVEMENT THERAPIST

Leading Clients to CORE Breath and Awareness

Noah Karrasch with
Robert White and Elizabeth Buri

Illustrations by Michael Eaton
Photography by Brian Holden and Komeil Zarin

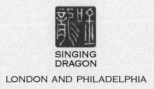

SINGING
DRAGON

LONDON AND PHILADELPHIA

Illustrations on pages 75 and 91 from *The Endless Web* by R. Louis Schultz and Rosemary Feitis, published by North Atlantic Books, copyright © 1996 by R. Louis Schultz and Rosemary Feitis. Reprinted by permission of publisher.

Image on page 98 from *The New Rules of Posture* by Mary Bond © 2006.

Reprinted by permission of Inner Traditions International and Bear & Company. www.innertraditions.com.

Photographs in Appendix A and B kindly provided by Behrooz Moshari.

First published in 2017
by Singing Dragon
an imprint of Jessica Kingsley Publishers
73 Collier Street
London NI 9BE, UK
and
400 Market Street, Suite 400
Philadelphia, PA 19106, USA

www.singingdragon.com

Copyright © Noah Karrasch 2017
Photographs copyright © Robert White and Elizabeth Buri 2017

Library of Congress Cataloging in Publication Data
Title: BodyMindCore work for movement therapists / Noah Karrasch with Robert White and Elizabeth Buri.
Description: London ; Philadelphia : Singing Dragon, 2017. | Includes bibliographical references and index.
Identifiers: LCCN 2016042911 | ISBN 9781848193383 (alk. paper)
Subjects: | MESH: Mind-Body Therapies--methods | Manipulation, Orthopedic--methods
Classification: LCC RZ401 | NLM WB 880 | DDC 615.8/51--dc23 LC record available at https://lccn.loc.gov/2016042911

British Library Cataloguing in Publication Data
A CIP catalogue record for this book is available from the British Library

ISBN 978 1 84819 338 3
eISBN 978 0 85701 295 1

Printed and bound by CPI Group (UK) Ltd, Croydon, CR0 4YY

ACKNOWLEDGMENTS

To all my students and teachers, on whichever
side of that fence you see yourself.

With special gratitude to:
R. Louis Schultz
Vivian Jaye
Jane Harrington
Emmett Hutchins
Wilhelm Reich
John Pierrakos
Stephen Porges
Peter Levine
Ralph Harvey
Mary Bond

Thank you from Liz:
Komeil Zarin, Photographer
Olivier DiTullio, Model and Tai Chi Guide

Thank you from Rob:
Brian Holden, Photographer
Kate White, my patient wife!

Contents

Disclaimer

This book features three authors; only one has a medical credential (Robert White, Chartered Physiotherapist). Our credentials all come from non-medical associations. Therefore, please take our ideas and advice in the spirit of exploration, not prescription. Ultimately, we all choose, somehow, our life, death, illness, or health. Others can assist us in directing that process toward wholeness, but each of us is responsible for finding our own answers. Those practitioners— medical and non-medical—who claim perfect healing every time from their services are charlatans. We strive to be better as we hope to help you become better.

"Go into the places where you hurt;
hopefully with someone you love,
definitely with someone you trust.
Feel the pain, listen to it, and then allow it to go away."

NOAH KARRASCH

Preface

This book began as an idea from Robert White, consultant physical therapist, Pilates teacher, and Level IV CORE bodyworker in Northeast England (www.body2fit.co.uk). Rob is director of *Body 2 Fit Ltd*—a physiotherapy, sports injury, and rehabilitation clinic. Several years ago he asked me whether we might create a book that presents CORE terminology and philosophy to Pilates instructors in a way that would empower them to apply those principles more fully in their own work. In the ensuing years as both of us have thought about such a book, we've realized that *all* movement therapists could benefit from our ideas...a guide to getting better results for clients by being more in tune with them, their bodies, and their restrictions up and down those client body lines. To do this we must get better results and clarity in our own practitioner bodies as well. The more we can help clients isolate, stretch, and release their restrictions (and our own), the less pain, the less lack of energy, the less curtailment of life happens. It's a worthy goal, and one we believe will be served by this book.

During the course of preparing for the writing, I invited another student, Elizabeth Buri from Malaysia, to participate in the writing as well. Liz is also a CORE Level IV worker, as well as a yoga instructor, Pilates instructor, and martial arts enthusiast (www.ourbodyspace.com). I believe, between the three of us, that we are able to offer valuable ideas that can both encourage and cross-pollinate any movement therapist to challenge their belief system and practice, opening their mind to new ideas and techniques across the spectrum of movement therapies. During courses with these two advanced students, I've often been pleased and surprised to find the inventive work they offer when giving movement cues to clients and partners in the work. I'm excited to mix traditional Asian influences with Western ideas in this book. With Rob's head, and with Liz's heart, my gut says we have a good book of challenges for movement therapists. And, as we finish the writing, I realize many bodywork therapists could benefit from incorporating more of this work into theirs.

About ten years ago I first started using the term "bodymindcore," which denotes to me that we can't just focus on a body. We must incorporate what's happening in the whole person...in the body of course, but also in the emotional, mental, and energetic states as well. To acknowledge only the physical part of any person without inviting them to examine their feelings, their feelings around their bodies, and their feelings around the pains and restrictions in that body, is to not treat the entire being. Some clients will resist the attempt to bring them into their full bodymindcore; it's still meant to be a goal of total healing. Too often clients want and expect us as therapists to "fix" them. This book challenges us to be better at involving the client more fully in their own process, and teach them how to "fix" themselves through movement work with a liberal dose of common sense. We all begin with bodies; how we choose to use them is where the variations occur. Can we all begin to use them more wisely, efficiently, and happily?

My CORE model is currently focused on the vision of four major centers in our body: head, heart, gut, and groin. In addition to these centers, I see gateways; between these centers as well as between the ground and groin, and between the head and heavens. It's my intention to help therapists learn to isolate their clients' trouble spots and provide helpful instruction as to how to release any restrictions in these centers and gateways so that energy flows freely through the entire being.

I trained as a rolfer in 1985–6. Prior to that time I was a musician and music teacher; working with and understanding rhythm, harmony, and melody. I've always thought that career helped me in this one... I hear and see the rhythm and melody of a body moving through space. But the *movement* of that melody, harmony, and rhythm becomes the joy of music, and of helping others feel better. Listening to only one note with no rhythm moving through would become boring and painful, just as no movement in life can become painful and debilitating.

From certification with the Rolf Institute in 1986 and advanced certification from the Guild for Structural Integration in 1991 I began exploring the concepts I advocate today. In about 1989 or 1990 I attended a Rolf movement workshop co-taught by Vivian Jaye and Jane Harrington. At the end of the six days of work (and probably at the beginning as well), both encouraged us to avail ourselves of Rolf movement work, *and* to become our own movement therapists, for self and for clients, if no registered movement therapists were available in our area. Ida Rolf's reason for asking students to develop positive movement work was that as we (rolfers) created better bodies for our clients, we also needed to teach those bodies how to move in this newer and better alignment. I accepted that charge and have investigated movement personally for all these years.

"Personally" means I've spent some time with movement experts: yoga and tai chi classes (no martial arts for me, though!), sessions with Rolf movement, Feldenkreis, Alexander, Pilates, and CORE Energetics practitioners, and dipping into many self-help movement books. Through all this help, and more, I've developed what works for me. I believe this is something we therapists must do for ourselves as individuals, in order to be our clients' most effective helper.

We want to coax them to develop the movement feel and style that serves them most efficiently as it invites them to explore and expand their personal core experience. And, if we're honest, most of us, like our clients, know what we *need* to do to help ourselves, but we only do it when we get into trouble!

So, though I consider myself primarily a bodyworker and teacher of bodywork, I also consider myself a purveyor of movement awareness to my bodywork clients, primarily through the filter of the learnings from my own body. These learnings were greatly accelerated by an accident in late 1987, only a year and a half after Rolf certification.

In that year many life changes had happened to me: newly certified as a rolfer, newly divorced, newly located to a new area, etc.—things were moving fast! In November, on the Thanksgiving weekend, a friend and I flew his two young sons in his private plane to Disney World in Florida for a short holiday. On his approach to refuel on the way home, he ran out of gas and had to set the plane down hard and fast on an Alabama city highway embankment. We were all injured.

His ankles were badly broken, beyond true repair. The children in the back seat had tucked into position and were only bruised and shaken. My spine was crushed and squeezed at L1; a compression fracture resulted from the impact of the seat belt stopping my forward progress. My spinal column was literally compressed into about 10 percent of its normal space. In addition my left leg was jammed into my body and paralyzed, and my head hit the dashboard at about 60 mph (96 km/h), opening a gash to the bone that required 30 stitches to suture back together. It was a tough and painful time, compounded by the fact that the first doctor I consulted told me, "It doesn't matter what we do with you; your nerves are dead, anyway."

After firing that doctor, I flew back home by ambulance plane, had surgery to repair the spine, and began a long climb, which continues to this day. When I finally walked almost a month after the accident, I looked a lot like Frankenstein's monster...external muscles hauled me around clumsily, while traumatized intrinsics tried to wake up again.

When I allow myself to think about it, I hurt. Much as I don't want to think about pain, I also realize if I don't think of it, acknowledge it, and ask it to change, I'll live the rest of my life hurting more and more as I get slower and slower.

That life-altering event has given me a blessing: I know I need to keep moving those places that don't want to be awake in my body, and I keep working at staying mobile. I've learned a lot about movement and the lack of it! Literally it took about a year to get my left leg up a step on its own power. My lower/mid back still gives me trouble from the spinal fusion and the Harrington rods installed, then removed a year and a half later per my request. I'm not in great shape, but, for the body I have and the injuries I've sustained, I'm in fantastic shape! I truly believe my movement awareness coupled with my interest in continuing to repair and reclaim has made the difference. I probably could have become a disabled welfare recipient, yet it never occurred to me to take that path. Instead, I was up as soon as possible, moving what I could, relearning how to walk, finding and soothing my jangled and screaming body parts, and navigating through life.

Rob's suggestion of a book for movement therapists therefore seemed like a great idea. I've lived a life of creating movement therapy for self and others, so it seemed appropriate to share ideas. The collaboration on this book hasn't always been smooth: we've irritated, misunderstood, and challenged each other as we refined our ideas and got on paper our most effective work in a way I believe has made for a better book. An example: I've nearly always removed the word "try" from Rob's exercises: "Try to visualize..." We either do or we don't. Working with others has taken a few more of my already disappearing hairs, but has made a better book, I believe.

So much of what I want to share in this book comes from that uphill climb; the struggle I've made serves me as I encourage others in their quest. I invite you, as a movement therapist or an interested reader, to consider the ideas I offer, along with those of Liz and Rob, and see if you can incorporate more bodymindcore awareness into your movement work with clients, and with yourself. Best of luck!

BodyMindCORE

The CORE® philosophy

I've based my bodywork on the image of the body as a six-pointed star, or even a starfish. I think the image translates easily to movement work as well. The points of this starfish are arms, legs, head, and tail. In this concept the core of the being (for me, the front, back, and center of the deep spine; one could argue inner arch to occiput, while others define core differently) gets too tight, thus pulling all the points deeper into that tight center. This tension causes a lack of circulation or energy; this lack of energy causes the pains we develop in response to stressors of physical, mental, emotional, chemical, electrical, or whichever *energetic* nature. As we open the center of this bodymindcore, we begin the process of allowing the entire star to unclench so the aches and pains of the restrictions can release and resolve.

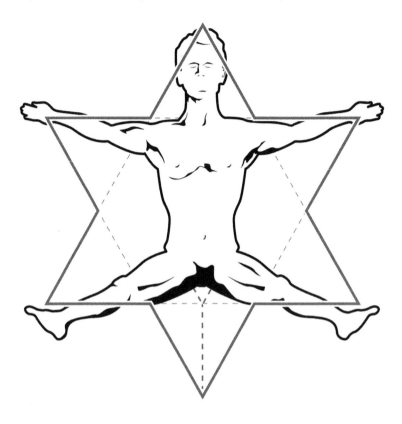

In this model I also see that, like a starfish's body, each of these six points has a bony prominence or skeletal point as well as a fleshy prominence or soft tissue or muscle point; the tip or end of bone and vein, if you will. The arm points end with the thumb bones and the fleshy thenar eminence, which is known as Great Eliminator (LI4) in meridian therapies; the feet have a similar configuration with the big toe bones and the Bubbling Spring point (KI) between first and second toes. The coccyx is the bony prominence of the tail area, and the genitals the soft tissue; their most prominent acupuncture point in this model is the Long Strong (GVI), between genitals and anus, near the coccyx. The cranial bones and the tongue form the last point of this star. A prominent point at the top of the head is GV23, also called the Upper Star. Any therapist in any discipline might well choose the goal of loosening that core experience so all six of those points could reach out into their world more fully and easily.

If we envision an elevator that runs through the core of our body, can that elevator move freely from and stop at every level of the body (including core but also arms and legs)? Or does it get "stuck" at one or more locations, ignoring other levels? This is critical in my worldview of bodies and the appropriate and necessary movement of energy through them...when we get stuck in certain parts of the body and ignore others, pain and dysfunction will result. Most of us are stuck somewhere in the middle—at the core.

Sometimes I wonder, as I compare my concept of a six-point star to the Judaic Star of David—was there some metaphysical significance to that symbol, now obscured? Does the symbol mean to challenge us to consider something we've lost? I further explore how one can subdivide that six-pointed star into its two triangles ascending and descending in bodies as well: The head point and the leg points form one triangle; the tail and arms/shoulders form the second. I often like challenging clients to stretch either of these triangles longer as well as stretching any and all points out of the core of the star. Though this "stretch" of the model doesn't work for all situations, it does make me more aware that I want to keep my eyes on the head when focusing on legs, or on the arms when working with the tailbone. Any stretch, in any direction, that encourages the points of the star to move further away from each other and from the core, is an appropriate piece of movement work.

So the goal of my work as a bodymindcore worker (which every good therapist from any school or technique may also adopt) is to open/lengthen/loosen the core of each individual I see, be it the Pilates core, a visceral core, my core, or some other model. How do we get people safely, happily, eagerly operating from a relaxed and resilient core? How do we get that tight, angry, or fearful something at the center of each bodymindcore to unwind and relax (not necessarily strengthen) while achieving a dynamic readiness and mutability that grounds and stabilizes that very operating system?

Then, how do we get all those six points of that star to further lengthen, open, unwind, and move forward from that core space... larger, in freedom instead of shortening back into fear? This is critical work in so many ways! I see the world as a place many of us are afraid of experiencing; we allow ourselves to live in fear and tension instead of enthusiasm and freedom. How can we open the points of our star when we're frankly doing all we can to remain tight and on guard?

The uncertainty of the world at the present time cries for a return to a feeling of individual core safety that we've long lost. How can we feel grounded when we're not sure we want to stay on this crazy planet? How can we live in a free and relaxed body when we're scared on the street, in our home, and on the planet far too much of our day? How can we move freely if we live with dug-in heels, girded loins, a stomach tied in knots, a tight ass, and a stiff neck? How can we coax our clients to find safety in such a state?

The CORE

This model builds on the concepts of many, including John Pierrakos, co-founder (with Alexander Lowen) of Bioenergetics. These two were the main disciples of psychotherapist and thinker Wilhelm Reich, who was years ahead of the field in his work on removing body or character armor and restoring the flow of energy through the bodymindcore. In Pierrakos' book CORE *Energetics,* he develops a model I've modified for my own understanding. Pierrakos saw humans as three-layered beings: their *core* is their *center of right energy*.[1] I envision not just the "Pilates core," which is usually identified by that group as something vaguely in the belly covered by a hyper-toned rectus abdominis.

CORE

Pierrakos saw humans as three-layered beings: their *core* is their *center of right energy.*

Mary Bond suggests that the true core is the site of our internal organs.[2]

Louis Schultz labels core as the body's central axis, though there is no structural correlate for this core.[3]

I see a vertical line that runs from the top of the head (and perhaps even above) and down into the ground through the feet at the deepest layer of our being.

All of us agree we need to move, spring, twist, and align from the core.

Pierrakos' next layer is the body, which needs no explanation, but is open to your speculation and understanding. Most interesting to me, he suggests the third layer of our being is outside the body: our environment. It's his contention that too many of us, in our desire to cope with the stressors of our world, use our bodies to protect our cores from our environment. I totally accept this model. Too many of us tense our bodies to withstand whatever life may be throwing at us, instead of allowing core self to flow into and through whatever experiences come our way, relaxing our body into acceptance.

We tighten

Muscles exposed to stress contract. When a bodymindcore experiences trauma, the body responds by contracting the flexor muscles located in the front of the body...we shorten and tighten the front of our cores. These contracted flexors inhibit the extensors located on the back of the body, in what we call flexor withdrawal. Unfortunately, most of us chronically live in flexor withdrawal. Situations that threaten us emotionally cause us to shorten and tighten our bodies in the same way that true physical threats will tighten us. The body will go into submission and withdrawal, slump and pull the head forward and down. Does this sound like many of us?

When we think of the current political, economic, and environmental situations in the world today (to name a few of our problems), we realize that, indeed, many of us are using our bodies to protect our cores from our environment. We'd be foolish not to do so! I'm interested in helping self and others find ways to stay in a relaxed and resilient body, even as we lodge on this unstable planet. How can we claim safety in our bodies when we feel unsafe in our environment? How can we have a body that shares with and shows its core to an environment it fears?

It's intriguing that psychologist Peter Levine, creator of Somatic Experiencing® (SE) work and author of *Waking the Tiger*, *In an Unspoken Voice*, and *Trauma and Memory*, suggests that the best psychotherapy in unwinding post-traumatic stress disorder (PTSD) involves keeping the client anchored in *body* sensations and feelings rather than the emotions. His SE work often takes a client into their traumatic experience, then asks, "What's going on in your body just now?" By keeping the client focused, in digestible doses, on both the trauma situation and body awareness, he's helping PTSD patients release that old trauma. He believes we heal from our pain and trauma when we face our fears, stay in our body, and learn to allow the fears to be seen and felt so they can be dealt with and moved through, into freedom.

Levine says that, "in order to experience this restorative faculty, we must develop the capacity to face certain uncomfortable and frightening physical sensations and feelings without becoming overwhelmed by them."[4] He suggests that too many of us move into *tonic immobility*, remaining stuck or frozen in a kind of limbo once we've been visited by a trauma. In other words, unlike lower mammals, we've lost the ability to shake out the fear and trauma from our bodymindcores. When that energy to the muscles is short circuited, potential energy becomes stored or filed as an unfinished procedure. Energy gets stuck.

On the other hand, John Sarno, a doctor of physical medicine, tells us in *The Divided Mind* that the root of many if not most illnesses is grounded in a wounded emotional state. He suggests **too many of us are in pain because we won't feel our feelings**:

> The true cause of pain, TMS (Tension Myositis Syndrome), serves the purpose of *primary* gain, that is, to prevent the conscious brain from becoming aware of unconscious feelings like rage or emotional pain... The ability to embrace sadness, hurt, or sorrow for oneself signifies a letting go of the self-critical aspect of one's personality and the development of self-compassion, which is a crucial ingredient for the successful reduction of psychosomatic symptoms.[5]

He believes we find it appropriate to hurt physically because we won't allow ourselves to hurt emotionally.

So from one perspective a doctor of the body invites us to open to our feelings and a doctor of feelings invites us to open to our bodies. Both see the importance of body and mind in relieving the issues of the core. I believe both are correct, as is Pierrakos; therefore we best serve when we get our clients involved in the full process—mental, emotional, and physical—to achieve true healing.

"Vaguely" scientific

Couple these leaders with a prominent researcher, Stephen Porges, whose book *The Polyvagal Theory* examines the role the vagus nerve plays in the ability of us all to remain balanced in our lives and world. The vagus is the only cranial nerve to descend into the body; it travels through the carotid channel and into the thorax where it autonomically enervates nearly all the chest, stomach, and groin cavities and their organs. The name itself means "the wanderer." The quote that most appeals to me from all of Porges' work is this one: "...the pivotal point is, can we get people to feel safe?"[6] Our vagus nerve is described by him and others as the "anti-anxiety" nerve. How can we feel safe if we feel anxious? Further, how can we create safety for our clients if they're in an anxious state, even as we're challenging them to examine their pains *and* their feelings? It's entirely possible that the best work we do with clients has less to do with teaching them how to move more effectively, and more about how to choose to live in their bodymindcores more fully, without fear of their environments.

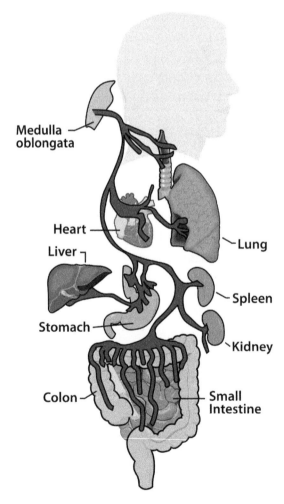

THE VAGUS NERVE COMPLEX AUTONOMICALLY CONTROLS
MUCH OF OUR BODIES' ABILITIES AND REACTIONS.

Porges has studied the vagus nerve for the past 30 years, and has helped lead us to new awareness of this little understood system. We're becoming more comfortable with the concept of the fight/flee/freeze system this nerve seems to evoke as it deals with the dangers of the world. Porges and Levine agree that we as a species need to learn "self-regulation." With this talent we would more quickly explore and examine the fears and feelings that come into our bodymindcore during danger and then choose how to process those feelings. We would move on through the trauma to the freedom and openness on the other side without the attendant tension and shortening of bodymindcore we so often develop and nurture. How can we, like our animal friends, face our dangers, decide how to act, and then move on through life without that situation's unprocessed information embedded in our tissues?

Porges tells us our earliest evolutionary nervous system hosts the "freeze" or play dead mechanism through the dorsal vagal nerve. This oldest mammalian network allows us to go into the default mechanism of freezing: shutting down and playing possum through our entire system when we feel our life is threatened. This system can also be called the "immobilization response." The secondary development of our vagus nerve is the "fight or flee" system of the sympathetic nervous system, which chooses how to *act* in any crisis situation. It's in fight or flee that we feel in danger and want to act. We've processed and decided we're not into shutdown, life-threatening danger, but we must still *do* something to survive. This fight or flee comes through the ventral vagus nerve. The third, newest, vagal development is the social communication and engagement system—that which can stop, look, reason, and choose another action, always maintaining our safety. This system is dependent on myelinated fibers of the vagus coming from the nucleus ambiguus in the brain, allowing us to process and decide how to act so the trauma doesn't get trapped in us. The parasympathetic system fosters calm as it exerts influence on the entire vagal system, tamping down the survival messages. It allows us to face and feel instead of fighting or fleeing.

In a healthy body system, we maintain balance between this older sympathetic nervous system that tells us we've got to do something (play dead, retreat, or attack), and the parasympathetic system that tells any of these responses to calm down because things are under control. When the vagus is stimulated and we believe we've got to take action, the parasympathetic usually kicks in to tell us to relax when the crisis is past. Unfortunately, for too many of us, this no longer happens—we get stuck in freeze, or fight, or flee. This ability to resiliently allow the parasympathetic system to bring us back "down" seems to dictate how we find health. When we find this resilience, we can self-regulate and return to balance; if we can't find balance, we suffer, as we're stuck in fight/flee or freeze. When we can't find this resilience, we get sick. We hurt.

One could see the sympathetic system as the gas of our vehicle; it lets us know we must make movement, and fast, in order to survive. If that's true, the parasympathetic system is the brake— that which tells us to relax and allow life to move forward at a moderate speed. Unfortunately, too many of us are running with both brakes and gas at full strength, too much of the time! When our vagus races due to danger, our parasympathetic system kicks in to dampen that gas pedal. Unless our sympathetic gas can slow down, we're choosing anger, depression, a racing heart, and a host of other unhappy circumstances. We're even finding that a new treatment modality involves implanting a sort of "pacemaker" that keeps our parasympathetic system on the rise, thereby allowing the sympathetic system to relax and lessen the severity of several medical conditions including arthritis and other inflammatory issues.[7] As we do relax, either we decide the danger is past, so the brain's amygdala sends signals to the rest of the body to return to calm, or we continue to perceive the danger and tell the bodymindcore to take action. It's continually answering the question "Am I safe, or am I at risk?"

Postural balance

Osteopath, author, and teacher Leon Chaitow states in Mary Bond's book *The New Rules of Posture* that, "Although there are sometimes structural reasons that prevent balanced posture and good use of the body, most of us are guilty of misusing our body machinery due to habit."[8] He sees a direct relationship between posture, pain, habits of movement, and the aging process we all endure, either gracefully or poorly, depending on our success with posture and movement habits. And let's add in Pete Egoscue, physiologist, who suggests in *Pain Free Living* (see Chapter 2) that postural balance can both calm the mind and beneficially affect our physiological systems as well.

So, Egoscue invites us to examine our posture. Chaitow tells us we misuse our bodies in ways that harm our posture and movements. Sarno suggests all our physical problems come from our emotional responses to our stressors. Levine shows how we move into freeze/flee or fight instead of feel. Porges believes we've all overstimulated our vagus nerve, and Pierrakos contends we're using our bodies to protect our cores from our environment...all tell us the same thing! *How do we get our clients to stand tall and move and breathe more fully from the core?* If we're going to get better, and to get better at getting others better, we've got to get more honest about the connection of the mind and emotions to the health and posture of the entire being.

Ida Rolf, PhD, developer of the Rolf method of Structural Integration, passed from this life in 1979 and I didn't connect to the Rolf Institute until 1984, so I missed her by a few years. I received much of her guidance through Emmett Hutchins and Peter Melchior, both of whom offered us her pearls of wisdom in their courses. One such pearl from class notes has been coming back to me a great deal lately: "Maturity is the ability to discern finer and finer layers of distinction." I believe she suggested to us that true maturity means we can slow down, and allow ourselves to look, feel, experience, and decide how to process, deal with, and eliminate each input from our environment without deciding to shrink, hide, or in other ways choose to tighten that core, lock down that body, and protect ourselves against that environment. We become mature when we allow ourselves to explore our world of thoughts and feelings instead of hiding from it.

So this book is offered as a challenge to movement therapists to get better at taking into account not only movement patterns and restrictions, but *any* restrictions which present themselves during sessions: The emotional and energetic restrictions are as important as, and possibly in many instances more important than, the physical problems that are manifestations of that emotional, psychological, and energetic pain too many of us hold in our physical beings. And possibly the most important lesson we offer: Creating breath awareness. We'll visit the need for better breath technique frequently in the coming chapters. Let's take a breath and activate our parasympathetic system, self-regulate, and move forward.

- I've based my bodywork on the image of the body as a six-pointed star.

- Any stretch, in any direction, that encourages the points of the star to move further away from each other and from the core, is an appropriate piece of movement work.

- Too many of us tense our bodies to withstand whatever life may be throwing at us, instead of allowing core self to flow into and through whatever experiences come our way, relaxing our body into acceptance.

- Psychologist Peter Levine suggests that too many of us move into tonic immobility, remaining stuck or frozen in a kind of limbo once we've been visited by a trauma.

- "...the pivotal point is, can we get people to feel safe?"— Stephen Porges

- How do we get our clients to stand tall and move and breathe more fully from the core?

2

Pain and the Brain

That tricky pain scale

It's an interesting concept to ask clients to rate or number their pain on a scale of one to ten, with zero being no pain and ten being unendurable tension. Some clients will tell us they're living in a number 12, yet they were smiling and laughing 30 seconds earlier! Others will give a number three when they're clearly in agony with every step or breath. Learning to translate their signals can become fascinating and humbling work, and a study we could all pursue more fully. Learning to help them face their pain and their brain can be a challenging but rewarding part of our sessions.

When I personally consider this pain scale, a number one suggests to me that 10 percent of that sufferer's energy is being used to cope with pain; a four suggests 40 percent, and so forth. How can someone be giving 120 percent of their energy to pain? Yet perhaps that's exactly what's happening for some of us. I remember a client years ago—a young woman who enrolled in a pain management academy near my home, and working with me to make changes in her life. When I asked her what number on a scale of one to ten her pain registered, she told me she lived with a 13! I was amazed by this answer, knowing she'd driven herself to the appointment. I don't discount her feelings and perceptions, but I'm curious as to why some of us can live with pain and function while others can't seem to tolerate even a small dose of pain.

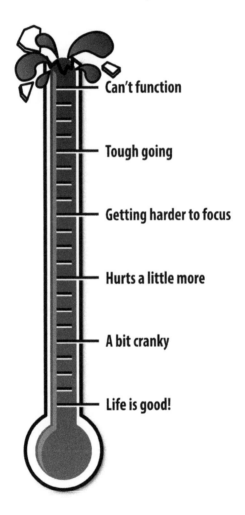

I've lived with pain and without; these days I tend to normally exist somewhere between one and two with spikes up to four or five occasionally, and that barometer seems fair to me.

Occasionally, 50 percent or more of my energy is devoted to pain management, and I can attest that it's not an easy life in the few times when that happens. After my wreck, when my number registered eight or nine, it was very hard to focus on anything except pain. I've had many injuries, and, when I overdo, either walking, standing, sitting, driving, traveling, or working too long and hard without attention to my own body's needs, I can make my own pain much worse, as many of us do too often when we tighten ourselves into a consistent non-moving or over-moving pattern to "power through" the pain. Generally I manage pain well and use only a small percentage of my energy to cope.

But how do we choose where we land on that pain scale? Do we choose? For some reason, some of us can live with a great deal of pain and make it be acceptable, while others live in a constant state of pain, making life difficult. Why?

What is pain?

Ida Rolf quotes Fritz Perls in (*Ida Rolf Talks about*) *Rolfing and Physical Reality*: "Pain is an opinion." Interesting concept! I think he suggests we can choose to feel or choose to transmute, but it's a thought-provoker.[1] In my student notes I also find she suggested: "Pain is resistance to change." There's something to consider here. The pain we're in is familiar pain, and the pain we might have if or as we let go of our known pain could be more severe. Therefore we often choose to remain in our comfortable, known pain. Too many of us are afraid to make that leap from the known into the unknown. Granted, Dr. Rolf was a pretty severe practitioner who actually probably created short-term pain in her clients in the attempt to free them from their anchored, long-term pain. These quotes make me think she expected her clients to yield to her ministrations without resistance.

Dr. Rolf's student and an anatomy and movement instructor at her Rolf Institute, Louis Schultz, suggested that pain is simply a signal that something isn't going right. If we think of pain as the cause of the problem, the logical response is to try to get rid of the pain instead of trying to locate the true source, face it, and release it. Egoscue suggests that pain is pain for a reason...it brings the bad news, so that it shouts louder than any other feelings we may have.

In one class I taught years ago to a group of massage students who primarily came from a nursing background, I mentioned the above Rolf/resistance to change quote. They immediately reacted: "Wait a minute! Pain is your body's signal that something is wrong!" After a moment of thought, I replied, "Could you say, then, that pain is resistance to something that's happening too fast?" They acknowledged that might be true. Pain is still pain, and still resistance, as far as I'm concerned. How do we help clients move into and through their pain, instead of allowing them to defend it more fully more of the time? This is critical in any therapy, and as movement therapists we have a special chance to take people into their pain, in acceptable doses, and ask them to explore and hopefully release and resolve that pain.

Recently a student gave me another insight into pain from something they'd heard; sorry to say, I can't source this idea: Pain is your body's perception that you are in danger. This seems to be an even better way to identify why we get into that fearful, "tighten up and stand your ground" kind of world... We feel danger, we want to protect our core from our environment, and we lock down the mechanism to feel secure. We tighten our cores to withstand whatever might come our way... We've dug in the heels, and we're ready. I've thought long and hard about that phrase that's all through the Old Testament of the Bible... Quite often God told the people to *gird their loins* because something catastrophic was coming. What does it mean?

I think the phrase's concept suggests tightening the core line as it relates to the earth. Specifically, I think we gird our loins when we ground ourselves into the earth by digging in our heels; then tightening the deep line of leg through tibialis posterior tissue, up into the girded thigh through adductor, and sucking that line up into psoas, iliacus, and quadratus lumborum as we reach up into the front of the spine...all the way up into the diaphragm cords and muscle, where we hold our breath as we tighten our core. If we tense that core all the time with girded loins, how can we ever get out of pain?

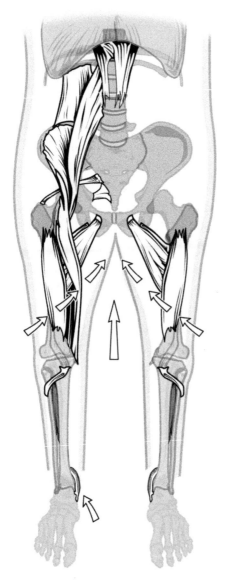

THE "GIRD YOUR LOINS" MUSCLES.

If we can meet our clients where they are, acknowledge their pain, listen to their story, and allow them to unwind their pain and their girded loins *while* getting breath through their being and helping them find their personal safe ground at a speed and depth they can tolerate, we provide them with a far greater service than just teaching them to move more effectively. If we push too far or too fast, we only create more pain and resistance. I've long told students in my bodywork courses that bruising simply means they've moved too deep and too fast. Most good deep tissue massage texts suggest the deeper we want to work with a client, the slower we must proceed. We can also push too deep and fast with movement cues or psychological cues. Simply by asking too much, we can cause clients to dig in their heels, re-gird their loins, and defend, instead of choosing to acknowledge their pain as a step toward releasing and resolving it.

Sarno, previously referenced for *The Divided Mind*, suggests pain is oxygen deprivation. When a tissue has a mild and localized reduction in blood flow to a small region or specific body structure which therefore isn't receiving oxygen, pain ensues. This gives us yet another reason to get clients breathing whenever we work with them! So, perhaps, instead of pain as resistance to change, pain could be seen as resistance to breath, to awareness, to learning how to live in and explore a tissue instead of blocking and congesting it. Sarno further suggests: "Almost all of the common pain disorders that have afflicted millions through the years are psychosomatic" (p. 45). Pretty strong words!

Sarno sees the drive to be perfect, or at least good, as the driving force in much of our pains. What he calls "perfectionism" and "goodism" are factors in the genesis of most pain...and many who are in pain are seen by him as victims of the pressures of life and the pressures they put on themselves. These feelings are derived, in his mind, from feelings of inferiority...feelings most of us have, if we're honest with ourselves. We create rage against these feelings of inferiority; as we won't allow ourselves to feel the feelings, we feel pain instead. He suggests almost all common pain disorders are psychosomatically based... We're in pain because we hurt emotionally.

"Pain is...

...an opinion."—Fritz Perls[2]

...resistance to change."—Ida Rolf[3]

...a signal that something is going on that isn't right."—Louis Schultz[4]

...pain for a reason...it brings the bad news, so that it shouts louder than any other feelings we may have."—Pete Egoscue[5]

...your body's perception that you are in danger."—Anon

...a response to an offense...[suggesting we] must have done something to cause the suffering."—Doug Nelson[6]

...resistance to breath, to awareness, to learning how to live in and explore a tissue instead of blocking and congesting it."—Noah Karrasch

...a gift if it's taken as a gift, or a curse if it's identified as a curse...that it's just the messenger!"—Noah Karrasch

Can we instead see pain as an opportunity to make changes?

Pain's messengers

Doug Nelson in *The Mystery of Pain* shares some interesting thoughts.[7] He offers that pain is a response to an offense (worked too hard, had a wreck, injured self, etc.), suggesting we've done something that causes us to need the suffering. Many of us still hold this or some such seed thought in our bodymindcores. Can we instead see pain as an opportunity to make changes? Can we let go of the notion that pain is the body's best and most effective long-term response to an offense committed against oneself? Perhaps this is sometimes true, but it's not always the case. Pain, from whatever source, may be useful, necessary, and possibly even life saving, but we must listen to its message to free it.

Our bodies have nociceptors, messengers which tell the brain "something" is happening; the amygdala in the brain interprets those messages and chooses responses. These nociceptors unconsciously tell us our environment sends stimuli which our brain interprets as safe, dangerous, or life threatening. Why do some of us have higher sensitivity and reactivity to those messages? Nelson suggests some of us have "hyper-excitable nerves." Turning down the volume, or inhibiting the nerve's response by artificial means (prescription medicines or nerve blocks, for example), very possibly won't work, because these interventions turn down the volume on the entire bodymindcore, giving us a less alive life. Yet, if we can't turn down this volume, we live in pain! How do we change the nociceptors' messages or find new messages so we can relieve the old pain?

And what do we do, once the pain signals are still sending even though the pain stimulus is no longer there? Chances are, we stay in that pain pattern. That old mammalian brain, the play dead mechanism, doesn't respond to pain mentally, but by changing heart rate, body temperature, and other essential bodily functions. The midbrain or limbic brain is the emotional center, and here is where we perceive our pain. The neocortex, the newer brain, allows us to think and plan. The midbrain and the neocortex seem to counteract each other...therefore, if we can activate our neocortex thinking brain and inhibit the midbrain's emotions, we can deactivate the emotions of pain, and the pain itself. The amygdala, in that midbrain, is currently the subject of much research into its function in creating and storing pain.

We're beginning to understand that, unlike ordinary memories, traumatic memories result from a breakdown of this system, such that the inhibitor nociceptors just can't keep up when our brain is processing in "trauma response" mode. In fact, people who live with

PTSD are shown to have shrunken brain areas of pre-frontal cortex, where self-awareness is processed, and in the insula where body awareness is processed. Trauma causes brain shutdown that needs to be rebooted. It seems our best reboot comes from allowing self (preferably with guidance) to simply observe these inner processes as they relate to the body while we relive, in small doses, the traumatic incident. With help, we can consciously rearrange our brain's perceptions of the trauma-inducing events and our response to them.

Fear and dread

Nelson suggests that we can think ourselves into pain, and that the *presence of dread* will substantially increase the presence of pain. He cites research that shows that learning to turn the mind to a new direction can also reduce pain. He suggests we learn to uncouple the emotion, fear, from the pain. By replacing the fear-emotion with something else, we begin to have a chance to create a new stimulus to the brain and a new conductivity away from the old pain. **We must learn to view the old painful situation dispassionately.** As fears diminish, pain subsides.

Egoscue says:

Fear is an extreme form of expectations... Being afraid is part of being human, and fear has its place in our emotional lexicon... Fear is particularly dangerous because it locks you out of the present moment and blocks the awareness you need to be in contact with your body... Fear may be the hydrogen bomb of our emotions: it's a last resort, an over-the-top response to an existential threat...we live in an era where the fear button is pushed again and again.[8]

Using this concept, it's easy to see why so many of us in this fear-inducing world live in pain.

Among the interesting research Nelson quotes, he reports that stress causes pain to register more severely, and that over-protective or over-sensitive parents produce children who respond to pain in a way that makes their pain worse! We can be conditioned to deal with and shake out pain, acute and chronic, or we can be conditioned to fear our pain and let it manage us.

Nelson also cites research that suggests we have an innate ability to shake out of the "freeze" mode, when we're paralyzed by our pain or fear emotion. Somehow we hit a reset button that allows us to move through the pain loop. This is important! If we can shake out that old painful traumatic event, either immediately after it's happened, or at some time in the future, we can release and resolve the painful messages. We want to learn to confront our pain as we become aware of the body *and* the emotions held in it. By staying with the message and getting a clearer picture of what our body is trying to tell us, then "shaking it out," we can also move through our pain. As Levine says, "Memory...chooses selectively from the past and builds on what was effective, while not repeating those responses that were deleterious or harmful."[9] Even as we work to remember and avoid anything that looks like a repeat of our old traumas, sometimes we only anchor them more effectively and fully. Among the simplest means of shaking out our pain response is a deep breath...slow, rhythmic breathing may be one of the single most effective ways to relax and let go of the trauma.

Move it; shake it out

So movement can be effective at positively changing pain and transforming, reducing, or eliminating it. An effective movement therapist helps clients create a better world for themselves; whether by this diminishment of pain, fear, and dread, or by an addition of joy, balance, and energy moving through their bodymindcore—movement works! And movement with breath, which we'll discuss soon, is even more effective.

Patrick Wall, a highly respected pain researcher and sometimes called the world's leading expert on pain, suggests that **movement is essential to pain relief**, so that any good work with pain reduction should incorporate movement work into any other form of treatment. I'd add to "movement" the concept of "breath" as well. Wall is perhaps best known for his "gate control theory of pain": We all have different sets of nociceptors, some designed to inhibit pain responses. If we can learn to manage that gate as we listen to those inhibitors more than those augmentors, we can decrease our response to the pain and feel we've decreased the pain itself.[10]

I have personal experience of this: After too much lifting, standing, bending, sitting, etc., I can find my pain scale registering "five." If I *stop, stretch and move, breathe,* and *focus on relaxing into the pain,* often I can recalibrate that pain to a "one," "two," or "three." Wall's concept of movement suggests that if and as we move, we're becoming more in touch with those inhibiting nociceptors that "take our mind off" our pain. Likewise, I add, if we can breathe into the pain, we further enhance the inhibiting signals instead of the augmenting ones.

So let's focus on the idea that pain can be a gift if it's taken as a gift, or as a curse if it's identified as a curse...that it's just the messenger! What we do with the message of pain is up to us. What we as therapists do with the messages our clients bring us must be done with respect, communication, and a bit of nudging that client to move into and through their pain if they want to move past it. Simple to say, not easy to do!

- The pain we're in is familiar pain and the pain we might have if or as we let go of our known pain could be more severe.

- "Could you say, then, that pain is resistance to something that's happening too fast?"

- If we hold that tightened core all the time with our girded loins, how can we ever get out of pain?

- Perhaps instead of pain as resistance to change, pain could be seen as resistance to breath, to awareness, to learning how to live in and explore a tissue instead of blocking and congesting it.

- Can we instead see pain as an opportunity to make changes?

- If we can activate our neocortex, thinking brain, and inhibit the midbrain's emotions, we can deactivate the emotions of pain, and the pain itself.

- We all have different sets of nociceptors, and some are designed to inhibit pain responses. If we can learn to listen to those inhibitors more than those augmentors, we can decrease our response to the pain and feel we've decreased the pain itself.

Partners in the Work

Communication skills and client participation are critical to good therapy! We don't "fix" clients; we offer them tools, awareness, and the opportunity to fix themselves. When we invite and coax clients to examine their own issues, keep them focused on their body sensations, and challenge them to remain in the sensations and stay in their bodies, we give them the opportunity to release and potentially resolve the issues they've been harboring. These issues may have caused them to live in a painful state and lose hope. We're all beings with a history; we've all got our story. I've been amazed to watch some people relive their old stories, again and again. If or when we start to help clients get better, some will continue to fall back on the old painful, yet comfortable, places because pain is what they know, and moving forward into something better might be uncomfortable to start. How do we convince those clients to move into the unknown or discard their old story and consider a new one? Posing a more basic question: How do we help clients *thrive* instead of merely *survive* when first they have to feel *alive*?

Talking the talk

Many schools of bodywork and/or movement don't teach communication skills; most medical schools certainly haven't caught up to the importance of learning to communicate clearly, honestly, and with compassion. Good talk therapists usually understand the value of communication skills, though some seem to listen far too little. Studies now show that doctors who demonstrate caring communication skills get sued for malpractice far less frequently, even when their mistakes are undeniable. If a client/patient/patron knows the risks of a procedure or treatment as presented by a caring "caregiver," they are far more likely to feel part of the process. By making the client or patient part of the decision-making process, all therapists are more likely to achieve success and less likely to be blamed for problems.

Research has shown that massage is rated more effective by clients if there is no extraneous talk; this makes perfect sense. However, massage is often performed with a goal of relaxation, and quiet makes sense for relaxation. But if we want to help our clients make changes, we're probably going to achieve more if we first listen to and validate their stories, then talk to them about what we're doing, why we're doing it, and how they can participate in the work to enhance its effect. If we can get them aboard with these ideas, in a partnership, more change will happen, and faster. This is true for movement work as well as bodywork; partnership is preferred to the model of expert and seeker, though some of us would love to think we are the expert.

Years ago a friend was serving in a responsible position in her local church. One Sunday, from the pulpit, the pastor announced that my friend had been replaced by someone new to the congregation. The pastor evidently felt the new convert needed a job to feel included. Without discussing first with my friend that this fellow was needy and there was an opportunity to plug him in while keeping my friend quietly in her position, the minister just dictated that someone new had the job. My friend was devastated! Shortly thereafter she left that church... Her reasoning seemed sound to me. She told me, "We all need someone to punch our ticket." When she felt invalidated by the minister, she had no more interest in being a part of the group.

This was an important lesson for me. Unless I can find a way to validate someone's feelings of pain, fear, and dread, and make it all right for them to have those feelings *even as they want to release them*, it will be much harder to help them remove such feelings and their manifestations. Looking back at Wall's gate control theory, does it seem that, in the desire to enhance the inhibitors in the new congregant, the minister caused pain in the established congregant by poking directly at her pain augmentors?

"Ownership" is a good word... **Can we first validate that client's pain or suffering or trauma?** Only then can we make them aware that they, or their circumstances, or their dread of their circumstances, may have contributed to or even created a situation or condition, and that examining that contribution is a fearless first step on the way to releasing it. We've all suffered through some good situations and some bad ones; suffering is the key. Was it really as bad as we made it? Once through it, do we continue to revisit it, and relive it? Or can we put the past in the past and learn to work forward from where we are into something more rewarding? Can we help our clients see that pain and trauma release is an act of forgiveness? Whether we need to forgive a person, a situation, a country, Mother Nature herself, or some intangible, we must learn to forgive the trauma that interferes with our living, breathing core.

Safe touch

Safe words and setting are important to any therapist as they communicate with clients, but tactile skills can be, and should be, just as important to movement therapists as their words and/or demonstrations are. Simple touch on a stuck spot or congestion, with continued request for breath and awareness, can change a pattern quickly and sometimes effortlessly. Too many movement therapists are shy of simple touch...yet touch is profound when applied cautiously yet lovingly, and with intention. Add to touch the concept of words that invite self-exploration: "What's going on in your body? What are you noticing right now? Is anything changing? What else do you notice? Are you breathing?" If words are effective, and touch is effective, how much more effective will we be if we allow ourselves to encourage words, touch, feelings, and partnership all at the same time?

Though I encourage movement therapists to experiment with adding touch to their sessions, it's not something I suggest is right for each of us. Some of us simply don't like touching; others will feel that, ethically, it's not in their realm. I/we respect these concerns. For that reason, we won't feature much hands-on practitioner work in the book (only a few *if assisting* cues from Liz in Appendix A). Props can be used for many touches—a bolster, a ball, a foam roller. Though touch can be effective, if one is afraid or shy about touch, allowing the tools to do the touching is perfectly fine. However, I do challenge all movement folks to consider being less afraid of touch and more willing to explore the profound changes that can occur with simple, effective touch.

Many of us will resist these ideas simply because we're not trained to be present for someone's physical or emotional breakdown. I'd argue: Of course we are! As caring people who acknowledge we won't judge another's path, but will give help where invited, I believe if we remain present with love, we are enough. I remember reading years ago in a book, "Where you are invited, you are empowered." It felt true then; it feels true now. When a client trusts one enough to break down and break through their overwhelmed state, that practitioner can simply be present, and if not validate, at least acknowledge without judgment, what one has lived through and in as they've tried to cope with their life's pain.

One of my favorite concepts in terms of successful therapies comes from *Persuasion and Healing* by psychiatrists Jerome and Julia Frank.[1] In this classic book, the Franks mention that their research shows four commonalities must be present for clients to heal.

First, clients must believe you care about them! Second, you provide a safe setting where they feel healing can occur. Third, you communicate your model, your goals, and your techniques to them. Fourth, you work in partnership and expect participation from the client. Instead of being the "doer," you are the team. I find this model to work tremendously well...the more I can make my patrons a part of the team where they feel safe and validated, where they understand what I'm trying to do and why, and where they want to help and participate to make changes, then changes will come.

Persuasion and healing

1. The client believes you care about them.

2. You provide a safe setting where they believe healing could occur.

3. You explain your model of healing to them, and why you think it's appropriate for their process.

4. You get the client on board as a participant instead of merely a subject.[2]

I've long used the concept of layers with clients and students. Layer one is that part of my bodywork, or any therapeutic session, where a client thinks: "This is delightful! I'm enjoying myself so much, and relaxing into this work." For me as a therapist, relaxation, while a worthy goal, isn't challenging the patterns at the root of the client issue. I don't often visit this layer. Layer two is the place where a client thinks, "What's going on here? Am I safe? Is this all right?" At layer two we're beginning to take the client into their vulnerable space where they have to choose to stay in their process, to go into their pain or fear so as to go through it.

At layer three we've lost them: They're now defending (fighting), running away (fleeing), or checking out (freezing). We've got to keep them in the present (feeling) mode if we want to help them move through their blocks. So layer one of therapies looks like fun; layer two looks like work; and layer three looks like a challenge too overwhelming. This overwhelm puts us deeper into our trauma, our loss of breath, our fight or flee or freeze modes, our pain. We as therapists can choose to refine our discernment so we can identify more readily on which layer we've got our client focusing their energy. Hint: The breath will tell you when you're too deep or fast.

Peter Levine in SE work uses the word "titration" to describe this condition. This old chemistry term suggests that adding too much of a substance may well cause an explosion! Proper measurement of the added ingredient ensures no such explosion occurs. This fits well with my layers concept...too much of a good thing is simply too much.

Reboot

Levine offers steps to renegotiating a traumatic memory. Though primarily for psychotherapists (though SE also trains bodyworkers and movement therapists), these steps offer cues as to how we can better help clients find their way through that memory and move forward:

1. Help create a here and now experience of a relative calm presence, power, and grounding.

2. Keep the client gradually shifting back and forth between the positive, grounded sensations and the more difficult ones (his term here is "pendulation").

3. Through sensate tracking, the traumatic memory emerges in the thwarted form that must be recognized and moved.

4. Having accessed, the therapist encourages further exploration of the senses associated and the development of the protections built around the traumatic experience.

5. This leads to a resetting of that core regulatory system.

6. The new memories are linked with and overpower the old traumatic experience.[3]

Once we understand the fight/flee/freeze/feel model, we can see how many people will try to escape or resist in some form or other—whether grinding their teeth while powering through (fighting), employing constant chatter or giggling (fleeing), or perhaps falling asleep or leaving their body (freezing): Chances are, any of these behaviors involves holding the breath while the body sorts out how to cope with the additional stimulus.

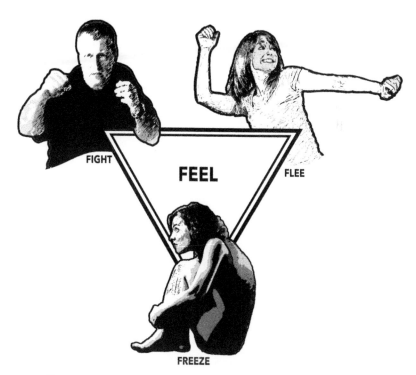

"WHERE DO YOU TEND TO RETREAT WHEN STRESSED?"

Can we as therapists get better at seeing where that client is stuck in fight mode, or fleeing, or freezing, and coax them to come out of their primary defense and move back into feeling, perhaps even neutral, instead?

Whether we're aware or not, movement should have sensation. Too many of us have discounted that sensation, which discounting hinders our movements. If we allow ourselves to feel the movement, we may feel the sensation, and we're not sure we want that. It can be upsetting to return to a feeling state. Physical or emotional threats cause us to shorten, tighten, defend, activate our sympathetic system, and shut down our bodies, depriving them of oxygen and causing pain.

Mary Bond in *The New Rules of Posture* seconds this idea. She believes movement is accompanied by sensation, felt or unfelt, within our nervous system...therefore, restoring articulation and movement can also restore sensation to our bodies. Some of us fight this restoration! "If you have ever felt shame or fear about any part of your body, you probably managed your feelings by withdrawing your awareness from that part. In effect, you made that part of your body disappear by immobilizing it."[4] And thereby, you created some of your own pain. She and others suggest that pain and limitation in the body aren't caused so much by the systems as the way we misuse them.

Coax

Most of us try to be perfect and good, which, while a worthy goal, really reflects our bottom line feelings of inferiority. Can you see how this perfectionism or not-good-enough attitude can cause us to further shorten, tighten, and stop the flow of energy through our body? We humans allow ourselves to become victims of our own need to do more and be better, and it's causing us to freeze within ourselves. Can we as therapists help coax clients into the realization that there may sometimes be a link between their pains and their self-denigration and need for external validation? Can we help them explore their feelings as well as their physical sensations? Can we help them decide the old story of who they are and how they feel, that they've habitually perfected and now stick with, is out of date, inappropriate, and ready to be discarded if they're going to be able to move forward and out of their pain and problems?

It's the practitioner's responsibility to keep that client in neutral feeling mode, with breath...*always with breath*, as they move into and explore their painful sensations and choose to evaluate and make changes in their world. Learn to talk to clients about what they want to change, keeping them focused on what's going on and what they feel as they move through the process. Help them explore the pain so as to identify and release. This is a skill many of us haven't developed. In addition to communication skills, we'll use breath awareness throughout this book as we work to enhance our effectiveness with our clients.

In that same vein, good work with clients involves the concept of coaxing change instead of forcing it. When we decide the client needs to change to meet *our* expectations, we become "the rapist" instead of "the therapist." This concept was pointed out to me by a damaged client nearly 30 years ago: It's still valid. In fact, I've even recently seen a cartoon with "The rapist" painted on a door in two lines, with a practitioner screaming, "It's one word!" When our need to change a client supersedes their need to change, we've taken their power and deprived them of the opportunity to discover their health.

Coax, don't force! I discovered rolfing and trained as a rolfer, a practitioner of structural integration, from 1984 to 1987. At that point Ida Rolf, founder of the work, had been deceased for about five years. The teachers I studied with continued to use her model of bodywork style, and it was pretty deep and brutal! In retrospect, I still believe much of the "emotional release" touted as a by-product of rolfing was simply a bit of overkill work. It seemed to me at the time we were pushing too hard and fast too often. Even in those days there was controversy as to whether rolfing had to be "hard," or whether "soft" rolfing could be as effective.

My personal answer is that both soft and hard work can be appropriate, but it's determined entirely by the client, the relationship of the practitioner to the client, the amount of trust that client has for that practitioner, and the client's desire to make changes instead of having someone else make the changes for them. Learning to "read" a client and their process and thoughts as one works with them will create far more effective work.

Effective and caring communication is a skill we could all develop more fully. If examining your communication skills to enhance your work intrigues you, please visit my book *Getting Better at Getting People Better*.[5] Meanwhile, just know that one doesn't go wrong learning to read the client bodymindcore more accurately, and learning to respond more quickly to the cues we see and sense.

- By making the client or patient part of the decision-making process, all therapists are more likely to achieve success and less likely to be blamed for problems.

- A good practitioner continues to remain focused on helping that client come into their present and look to the future instead of allowing them to remain stuck in their old stories.

- Simple touch on a stuck spot or congestion, with continued request for breath and awareness, can change a pattern quickly and sometimes effortlessly.

- The more I can make clients a part of the team where they feel safe and validated, where they understand what I'm trying to do and why, and where they want to help and participate to make changes, then changes will come.

- Whether we're aware or not, movement should have sensation. Too many of us have discounted that sensation, which discounting hinders our movements.

- It's the practitioner's responsibility to keep that client in neutral feeling mode, with breath...*always with breath*, as they explore their painful sensations and choose to evaluate and make changes in their world.

- In that same vein, good work with clients involves the concept of coaxing change instead of forcing it.

4

Life Is Easier with Breath

Watching the body to see where breath happens or conversely is being held can give any therapist important clues and cues as to what needs to happen to release and resolve stuck energy. In any type of therapeutic work, breath is, or should be, critical to success. Just as a psychotherapist monitors body signals, including but not limited to the breath, and a massage therapist notices lack of breath in their client and encourages fuller and deeper breath, movement therapists will enhance their clients' results by paying attention to and encouraging full, open breath, throughout the body. As Liz says later in the book, "Energy goes where breath goes. Movement goes where energy and breath go."

You've probably realized by this point in your career, even if you've only begun, how many people don't breathe well. When we ask for a deep breath, sometimes we don't even see movement of chest or stomach. A great part of our work is trying to get clients to realize they could breathe more deeply. Many of us were also trained as singers to keep our shoulders still with the breath. I see no reason to inhibit breath in any direction at any time. Breathe! And breathe as fully as possible, all the time. Simple attention to breath may be the most important cue we can give our clients. In my class called "The Top Ten Hot Spots to Effect Greater Change," the first place I want to touch a body is in the costal arch area, where I intend to create fuller and deeper breaths.

I'm intrigued how, more and more, we're realizing the effects of stress on our bodies, our minds, our bodymindcores. Although currently we're beginning to talk about positive stress, too many of us are living in a too-stressed environment that's taking away our breath! As we discuss vagus nerve, heart rate variability, and fight/flight/freeze, keep in mind that all these concepts relate to our stress levels *and* our ability to deal with those levels—to self-regulate.

A healthy heart

Current research on the importance of breath work indicates that heart rate variability (HRV) is enhanced by the simple mechanism of breathing in and out at roughly six times per minute (this varies between 4.5 and 7 for different people). This enhanced HRV, the change in the time intervals between adjacent heartbeats (meaning higher high speeds and lower low speeds in the rate of heartbeats), creates a greater spectrum in the breath mechanism, but healthier bodies as well. Enhanced HRV has been tied to such disparate factors in the body as improved immune function, less inflammation and arthritis, reduced cardiac problems, less diabetes, etc.[1]

Enhanced heart rate variability

- Improved immune function

- Less inflammation and arthritis

- Reduced cardiac problems and hypertension

- Less diabetes

- Reduced anxiety, depression, asthma

- Less SIDS (sudden infant death syndrome)

- Reduced gastrointestinal disorders

- Improved psychological resiliency and behavioral flexibility

All the above are shown to be enhanced by higher HRV.

"Vagal pacemakers" are now being installed in patients with arthritis and other inflammations; research projects are finding changes in HRV and healthier individuals from this direct vagal stimulation.[2]

In other words, by simply learning to breathe in at a slow and steady rate, clients are already beginning to heal themselves. This contributes to what I call the "vagal reset" and which Levine and others call "self-regulation." All of us suggest the client has remembered how to discharge the energy of the held breath, take the next cleansing breath, and reset the vagus nerve's system to return to the sympathetic/parasympathetic balance. As I call this vagus the "nerve of well-being," it makes sense that if we can reset the breath and the vagus, health is on the way. And it's intriguing that so far, the most effective vagal resets I'm aware of include deep bodywork, meditation, yoga, mindfulness practice, humming, singing, breath work, and *movement.*

Vagal tone is about balance—finding and maintaining it. The autonomic nervous system (ANS) controls the sympathetic nervous system (SNS) and the parasympathetic nervous system (PNS). The SNS gives us increased metabolic output in relation to the stressors we see coming our way, while the PNS usually promotes growth and restoration. In other words, the SNS senses danger, and it's up to the PNS to figure out how to tamp that danger back down, through self-regulation and after appropriate action, so the body can thrive. Balance between these two systems seems to be sorely lacking in many of us. Most of us have good vagal tone during rest, and that tone is actively withdrawn when we feel in danger.

This leads us back to the earlier concept of "vagal brake"...when we put on the brakes to calm the feedback that tells our body: "*Do something!*" Remember, our body is trying to apply gas and brakes at the same time. When we apply the brakes, our heartbeat also changes. Respiratory sinus arrhythmia (RSA) is the speed of heart rate, directed by vagal tone or lack of it. This RSA tells us whether our nervous system is working happily, and may even index an individual's true health or illness, as well as the ability to get the parasympathetic system under control so we return to neutral or feel state. RSA also relates to the above-mentioned HRV; they will work in concert or not, depending on our personal ability to self-regulate.

Fight, flee, or freeze?

Somatic Experiencing builds heavily on the idea that we have several vagal nerve paths, each having different mechanisms for dealing with life's challenges. Levine sees the *dorsal* vagus nerve as the older, reptilian, "play dead" or freeze mechanism of the body. In other words, if a threat is too great for a bodymindcore, the oldest effective method to deal with the threat is to simply play dead and shut down the mechanism. Consider an opossum, which is able to do just that. Other animals have the same talent: Mice, lizards, and other creatures can affect a death-like state until danger has past, at which point they "come to" and move on with their life. We humans also have this mechanism!

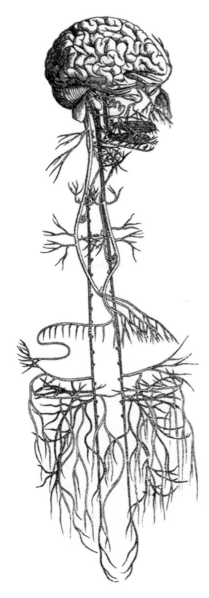

OUR COMPLICATED AND EVOLVED VAGAL SYSTEM.

As I think of this play dead idea, I realize many of us do exactly that: We skate through life, don't engage with others, don't allow ourselves to feel our feelings, and become "dissociated" from life itself. Playing dead is an old coping skill—maybe our oldest. While it might be effective in certain life-threatening situations, it probably isn't the most efficient way to go through life today. Part of the antidote is simply remembering to breathe again! Recognizing that the sympathetic nervous system has returned to one of the oldest survival mechanisms in the body allows us to return to simple focused breathing. We can activate the parasympathetic nervous system and self-regulate our body's survival responses if we can breathe well.

The second evolution in the nervous system, the activity system, is the sympathetic system's fight-or-flee response. This *ventral* vagus nerve lets us choose which of those actions seems more appropriate. Do we gird our loins and go into defense, then attack? Do we stand and fight, or do we run away instead? Many of us seem to be stuck in the fight system, and tend to make life one big wrestling match. Fight can be an appropriate choice, but constant on-guard behaviors will absolutely wear us down and eventually cause pain. Others choose to run away from whatever the threat may be; they'd rather simply ignore the problem by removing themselves from it. While similar to playing dead, when running away we're not dead; we've just autonomically moved to someplace that feels safer. In either of these mechanisms, the breath is inhibited to save energy for the fight, or for the flight. Eventually we'll remember to breathe again (hopefully!)...but first, we hold our breath as we sympathetically activate, then choose which behavior will be most appropriate for the situation. Again, can we reactivate the parasympathetic system and self-regulate our body back into alert rest, with breath?

Think of the medical diagnosis fibromyalgia. We have tests to determine if someone has the condition. If we find they do, we may give them a chemical substance to help control it, often with little success. I believe fibro is simply a condition of being traumatized and remaining stuck in that traumatic feeling, not being able to reclaim breath. In this situation as in many others, breath needs to come first!

Feel, face, and find freedom

The third and newest vagal system is the *self-regulation* system—what I think of as the "feel," or perhaps "friendly" or "face it," mechanism. This system is composed of myelinated nerve fibers that allow us to process instead of go into default mode. This evolutionary step allows us to think, to reason, to choose a different and better behavior. We don't have to live in a no breath, no life situation where HRV has shrunk because we're too focused on staying alive and negotiating our unfriendly environment in sympathetic mode. It's only when we use our ANS chronically for defense that we begin to have dysfunction and disorder in our organs and bodies.

The primary question for movement therapists and any other therapist as well is: ***How do we keep that client in their "feel" or "neutral" mode while they're breathing?*** And, as we remember Wall's idea that if we can replace the pain presenters by enhancing the pain inhibitors, we can help clients resolve that pain. Can we see that movement, breath, our presence, and the client's desire to change can make great differences? To be more effective we become better advocates for that client learning to:

- enhance HRV with their breath.

- self-regulate their sympathetic/parasympathetic balance.

- move through fight, flee, or freeze and back into feel or neutral.

The overriding questions of this book therefore may be: How do we free clients from their freeze, fight, or flee behaviors and keep them breathing into their neutral feel mechanism? How do we help them view and evaluate whatever comes into their world, and make appropriate decisions to process and eliminate the stimuli of the environment, instead of storing those stimuli in their bodymindcores? How do we get them to realize they've become stuck in their modes and their stories? How do we get them to breathe, shake out the trauma that caused them to gird their loins, and move on into and through life?

Louis Schultz says this well in *The Endless Web*: "We're not taught to walk as children, and we're not taught to breathe. The most common tendency of anyone frightened is to hold his or her breath... Holding the breath is a way of stopping that physical flow. Perhaps we do this because we don't want to experience the sensation of the emotion."[3]

I suggest clients learn to breathe in for a count; whatever count they can find, I challenge them to expand that count by a bit. Then I ask them to exhale to a slightly longer count. It's reasonable to assume that a slightly longer out-breath will assist in the cleansing of the lungs, removing some of the "stuck" energy therein, and replacing it with cleaner oxygen. I think it's also a good idea to ask them to have a short pause between inhale and exhale, simply to allow for a rest and reset of the entire system. Remember our earlier discussion of heart rate variability and the research showing that about six breaths per minute can enhance HRV, and thus contribute to a healthier body? It makes sense to teach clients to take longer, slower, and deeper breaths.

I also use breath as an assessment tool; I find noticing where a client's breath won't move often gives me clues as to where I should focus my work. Probably you've already noticed this phenomenon: Can you harness your observations so as to add one more tool to your toolbox as you assess, listen, communicate, and get participation from your clients, on their way to restoring their breath? Personally, I watch the breath a great deal; when I see breath lifting the shoulders naturally and not forced, and even reaching the head, I can tell we've made progress. Generally the client will feel that change at the same time as I see it. Often the breath will make small "jumps" when they've opened a new or formerly closed area of their body. So I perceive energy as breath flow.

A practitioner of any work can learn to observe, "ride," and encourage breath; a bodyworker can learn to apply mild brakes on an in-breath and gently nudge a bit deeper on the out-breath. A movement therapist can learn to coax clients into fuller breathing patterns, expanding breath awareness into painful and stuck spots of the bodymindcore—places clients don't necessarily want to visit. A psychotherapist can monitor breathing to see how painfully embedded issues are stored in the client's tissues as well. Attention to breath is always appropriate, and will be brought up throughout the book! Simple question: As you read this passage, are you breathing? Of course the answer is yes; the better question is, how deeply? How effectively are you breathing? Are you enhancing HRV, or just getting by in a fight, flee, or freeze mode?

- So far, the most effective vagal resets I'm aware of include deep bodywork, meditation, yoga, mindfulness practice, humming, breath work, and movement.

- Playing dead is an old coping skill—maybe our oldest.

- Do we stand and fight, or do we run away instead? In either of these mechanisms, the breath is inhibited to save energy for the fight, or for the flight.

- How do we keep that client in their "feel" or "neutral" mode while they're breathing?

- How do we get them to breathe, shake out the trauma that caused them to gird their loins, and move on into and through life?

5

Energy Work, Seen and Unseen

Whether we believe in the concept of energy work or not, we are energy workers! Call it energy, call it chi, prana, circulation, or oxygen, blood, or nerve movement...energy is there, even if it's inhibited. Sarno tells us that when energy or oxygen doesn't move through the body, pain results. The more we restore circulation as practitioners, the less pain our clients will hold in their bodies. So we needn't discount the concept of energy flow; we just need to choose words we can feel comfortable using, and introduce our clients to concepts that make sense to them. Just as I honor a client who tells me I'm digging an old spear or knife from a past life out of their shoulder, whether I accept reincarnation or not, each of us has our particular model of what life and its energies are about. As therapists we can validate that client and their model, whether we share it or not.

In the first chapter I mentioned my image of the body as a six-pointed star, with arms, legs, head, and tail as the starfish's points, and alluded to the acupuncture points near the ends of each extremity. The Bubbling Spring and Great Eliminator complete the hands and feet; the Upper Star at the head and the Long Strong near the tail and perineum also show us how these points are important to health function, just by their names. The Chinese medicine system has been successfully propagating wellness for thousands of years, based primarily on this model of moving static energy. The Chinese see all their meridians flowing up and down the body—one into the next in a continuous loop of energy. It's the treatment goal to move this energy through stuck spots on any meridian, often by applying needles or pressure either above or below the inhibited area. It's worked for a long time, so why discount energy?

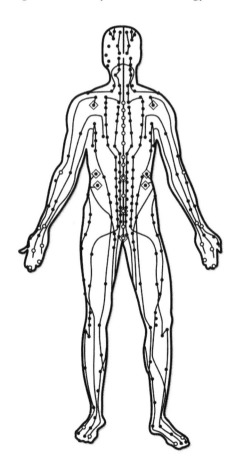

Energy sensitivity

Some people have greater energy sensitivity and some less. The fact that I can't see and feel energy in the way others who practice various healing modalities can do, or that I have a different belief system, doesn't mean that energy flow or lack isn't there! As we accept the concept that there is a flow or a lack, part of what we're trying to do is restore that flow. If we do so, clients will improve, particularly when we listen to and respect their model and their values.

Energy =

- Circulation
- Life force
- Chi
- Prana
- Blood flow/circulation
- Nerve conductivity
- Oxygenation
- Communication
- Movement

I used to be quite suspicious of "energy workers," and some still arouse my suspicions. I've personally had some profound healing experiences at the hands of energy workers as well as having felt no change whatsoever from others. I believe other factors are involved in the energy exchange. For example, some people don't attract me for various reasons. I'm less inclined to trust someone who demonstrates either a terrific ego or absolutely none as much as I'd trust a more balanced-seeming person. Just as I'm less interested in a practitioner who smokes cigarettes because of my "gut" reaction, sometimes my gut either really resonates with an energy worker (or anyone else) and sometimes it really clashes with something about that person—something energetic.

In a previous chapter I cited caring, providing safety, explaining the model, and getting client participation as four pillars of sound therapy. It's hard for many energy workers to explain their work. Yet if clients have no rationale for what's being done, they're less likely to see a positive outcome. I remember one chiropractor who used to work in my town. Clients never realized she did all her work based on what her small pendulum was telling her as she worked sitting above their head where she wasn't seen as they lay on her table. Had many known what she was doing, they wouldn't have stayed! But as she quietly employed energy forces and talked about her chiropractic work instead, and results happened, she was quite busy.

As movement therapists we are doing energy work whether we know it or not. As you care and create safety, your energy is doing the work. As you explain the work and get the client working with you, energy is exchanged. So, you are an energy worker! Being aware of this truth allows you to shape your energy work into more effective movement therapy.

Energy is life

Here's an interesting quote from Pete Egoscue in *Pain Free Living*: "We are energy. Our understanding of physics tells us that energy is indestructible."[1] Physics teaches us that every living being, but also things we consider to be static and "dead," have energy...the more static an object, the slower the movement of energy. Yet even rocks have energy! Some of our clients have turned into rocks; it's our job to help the energy move through them. If the model of energy movement doesn't work for you, find words and descriptors that do work, so you can bring your client along in this "energy" work. Choose a way you can allow yourself to believe in that energetic flow and look for it in your clients. Do you see changes in skin color or texture? Do you notice a general relaxation of the body? A deeper, cleansing breath and exhale? A spot where nothing seems to move? An imbalance side to side on the body? A twitching of an extremity? A feeling of loosening of tight tissue, *somewhere*? All these various observations can tell you energy is moving more fully or where it's still constricted.

Also, allow intuition to be present as well as science. Many people live in their heads, and expect to learn a protocol that will cure what ails the client 100 percent of the time. Yet no such protocol exists because each client on their personal journey has a different configuration of restrictions from anyone else who comes through our door. We are like snowflakes; no two are alike. Dependence on a protocol prohibits the practitioner from using their intuition, which is a valuable tool. While intuition is obviously not 100 percent foolproof, those who learn to trust their intuition and explore where it takes them can have remarkable results with clients as they follow their hearts while remaining aware of the head's messages as well. Malcolm Gladwell in *Blink* cites research showing those who seek too much information actually make less effective decisions than those who grasp the major concepts of a situation, then go with their gut![2] We can get so far into our heads that the rest of the body doesn't get a vote; can we use the head, but also the heart and gut, as we work with others, and ourselves?

Dr. Rolf used to say, "When you try to fix symptoms, you'll get into trouble." Unfortunately this is true too often. Our heads want to fix others even while our hearts simply want to support them. While many times symptoms disappear as we simply work to align a client in gravity and get breath and energy flowing through them again, too often we allow ourselves to chase down the rabbit hole of symptoms. We then end up in a Wonderland where we've unwound the presenting problem but unwrapped a whole new bundle of yarn that now needs to be unwound. Stay with the concept of balancing a body and enhancing energetic flow through that body by looking for and resolving stuck spots. This model seems superior to allowing self to get mired in what I think of as paint-by-number therapy. Interestingly, the longer one works to align clients in the gravitational field and enhance the energy flow, the more symptoms resolve themselves, and more quickly.

As we proceed with the book and my ideas about good movement work, it becomes clearer to me that there are often unseen, esoteric energy lines...some of us do see them! Others feel them, and others can rationalize how they might be present. With whichever tools you work, imagine that what you're doing with the right toe is traveling in the direction of the head and neck, or the same side or other side arm and shoulder. Begin to allow yourself to realize energy travels from every part of the body to every other part in a healthy and balanced individual, and can get stuck or slowed, causing an individual to lose that healthy energy flow. Begin to imagine where the energetic blockages up and down a client's body may be restricting that flow, or where pain is "growing" in response to such blockages. Allow yourself to expand your model of energy and you'll be rewarded with new knowledge.

So whether you as a practitioner live in your head, needing protocols and specific techniques, or whether you totally trust your intention, disavowing the need to have a formula, I'd invite you to consider softening your edges, and learning to call on both intelligence of the mind but also intuition of the heart and gut. Energy is real, whether we sense it or not. As we allow that reality, we become more sensitive to energy or its lack in the bodymindcore. As we become more sensitive, we become better practitioners. So, explore energy!

- As movement therapists we are doing energy work whether we know it or not.

- Choose a way you can allow yourself to believe in that energetic flow and look for it in your clients.

- Stay with the concept of balancing a body and enhancing energetic flow through that body by looking for and resolving stuck spots. This model seems superior to allowing self to get mired in what I think of as paint-by-number therapy.

- Allow yourself to expand your model of energy and you'll be rewarded with new knowledge.

6

Stretching the BodyMindCORE

Let's add a very important part of movement work to the breath, communication, and energy—the stretch. It's an ongoing debate with current research as to whether static stretches or moving ones produce better effects with less injury. I've found that moving stretches—even mild ones—*with breath* involved fully are most effective in getting clients to move through their blocks. I argue that the breath *becomes* the movement; if breath reaches an area, that area is stretched. If breath doesn't attain an area, tissues are static and remain blocked. Going back to previous chapters, can one also see how holding the breath enhances the pain and therefore deprives the body of oxygen, thus creating more pain?

I've long used the image of a rubber band with clients and students: If one holds only one end of an elastic band, little stretch can occur. If one holds both ends and pulls apart, a satisfying stretch occurs. If one twists those ends, puts a foot or some other blockage at the middle of the elastic, and moves it away while twisting and pulling, yet more directions of stretch are found. This is crucial to getting maximum work accomplished in a session. One can nearly always create another direction added to a stretch to enhance its effect. Once one accepts this simple idea, possibilities are endless in terms of coaxing clients to find disparate parts of the body that may be joined too tightly, and asking for stretch between them.

In Appendix A we three will offer, as a reference, cues which support finding, releasing, and resolving problems or stuck spots in each of the centers and gateways we'll explore in Chapter 8. We'll create simple and effective ways to help therapists show their clients more fully how they can move and create awareness in their own stuck spots. In Appendix B we'll explore further by working with this rubber band model; instead of focusing on one spot up or down the bodymindcore chain, we'll challenge therapists to help their clients realize how the tension in the ankles contributes to tension in the head or heart centers; how releasing the neck can contribute to opening in the pelvis. We'll see the body as a long elastic band that's gotten brittle, stuck, and lost its resiliency. We'll work to restore resilience through the entire line of the body.

Our "personal line"

For several years I've used the term "personal line." Basing my model largely on the pioneering work of Louis Schultz, Rolf Institute faculty member, anatomist, and author of *The Endless Web*, I've developed my concept that each of us has a personal line of transmission, with one or more blocks or congested spots that keep us from realizing our movement potential and therefore keep us from true health. Louis used to ask us as students to "go from the left ear to the right big toe in as few muscles as possible." I believe he was challenging us to simply be aware that there always is such a line of transmission.

Let's detour into Louis and his work, as he was definitely a pioneer in the fields of fascia and movement. Louis served as anatomy, movement, and assistant instructor in my Auditing phase of Rolf training, in early 1986, co-teaching with Stacey Mills. He was my introduction to many important ideas. Retrospectively, I realize how much I owe my style of work to nuggets that Louis tossed us in that course:

- (to clients and students): "What you're doing is good, *and* you might want to try..."

- (to students): "Give clients one or two movement cues—not three! They'll forget everything if they're overloaded."

- (to clients): "Now, go home and *play* with these ideas."

- (to students): "See each chakra as aligning with a diaphragm of the body as well." (The illustration from *The Endless Web* on page 75 gives an indication of these.)

- (to students): "Trace a line from the left ear to right big toe in as few muscles as possible."

- (to students): "I had trouble with Ida Rolf's concept of a Line until I realized that line could be flexible, like a fiberglass fishing rod."

- (to me personally, on receiving work from him): "Get out of your effing head!"

Movement and posture

In addition, movement-wise he gave me/us several other gems to ponder and polish with the passing years. First, touch is fine for a movement therapist if you are in the appropriate space and stay clinical. I watched Louis working very near a woman's groin, but she didn't feel violated at all, due to his professional nature. If you can't get comfortable touching, you probably shouldn't touch...but if you can be professional, so much more will be accomplished! Second, Louis told us the attitude of flexibility is important! When we consider our Lines to be flexible rods, instead of something that must be upheld perfectly vertical all the time, we can live in a comfortable body, resiliently. And finally, it's okay to be radical in your body at times, if you can find neutral when it's time to take off the high heels, or step away from the computer or out of the car. If and when we can learn to seek, find, and enjoy neutral more of the time, we can stay in a happier body as well.

Another quote from Louis:

> Movement can be evaluated from the outside by a trained observer. It is evaluated from the inside by proprioception. This is the internal physical sensation of position in three-dimensional space. Most of us can sense our bodies to some degree. When we tune in, however, it is surprising how many parts of our bodies we don't feel... When we talk about movement we usually think of large gestures like walking, doing work, picking up the baby, washing the dishes, driving the car. Yet movement can be as subtle as slow breathing during sleep. A body never stops moving. Even the smallest movement creates a ripple throughout the entire organism. The tissue through which this ripple is transmitted is the connective tissue.[1]

I've always thought of Louis as an underrated genius and am glad *The Endless Web* is seen as a classic introduction to connective tissue or fascia. One of his more important contributions, besides bringing Ida Rolf's speculations and his own conclusions about fascia (connectivity, conductivity, resilience, and support) into our discussions and awareness of its properties, is his chart of restrictive bands that show some pretty universal body problem spots. He doesn't suggest all of us have all this tension, but encourages us to look for such holding patterns as we chase those fascial planes from ear to toe.

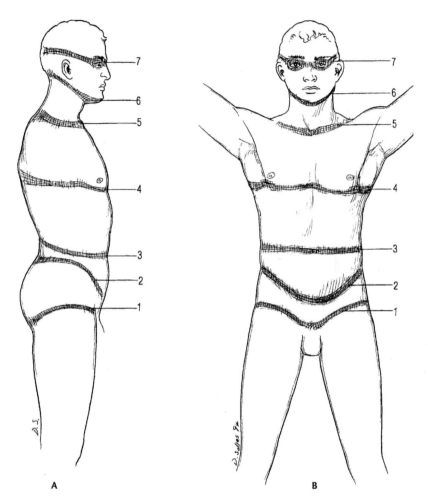

A

B

SCHULTZ'S MODEL OF FASCIAL RESTRICTION BANDS...
DO YOU SEE A SIMILARITY TO CHAKRAS?
Source: From Schultz and Feitis, The Endless Web, *p. 55*

Rolfer Mary Bond in *The New Rules of Posture* sees posture as something that's also moving—a new concept for many of us!

I see posture not as how you hold your body when you're still but as how you carry it while you're moving. This distinction reveals posture to be a dynamic activity rather than a static attitude. Your posture is generated by your movement... How we stabilize ourselves determines our posture and the freedom, efficiency, and grace with which we move. The essence of posture, then, is the unique way in which each of us negotiates between moving and holding still in relationship to gravity.[2]

Interesting distinction!

Mary has two simple rules for good posture: First, turn to self-study of your own posture and create a new sense of what feels balanced and stable (this will take help). Second, remember that posture is dynamic and moving, not a static something that you can plant and forget. It's an ongoing perceptual process in which you orient self to gravity and the bigger universe—I suggest, Pierrakos' "environment."

One of the reasons we suffer more in this modern age is that we've become less physical in our work and play...with tool-making we first learned to reduce our efforts. Where we used to move physically all the time, these days, more of us sit: in a car, at a computer, in front of a television. How can we be healthy if we're static? Ida Rolf always suggested that horizontality was the least efforted posture; standing was next. Sitting was the worst posture we could maintain. These days we're even likely to read articles and see research telling us that sitting is the new smoking. Sitting is indeed a tremendously difficult posture to maintain, and we're all required to maintain it more and more of the time. No wonder we hurt!

About fascia...

I often talk to clients and students about connective tissue as I try to bring them into my worldview of how we're living in our bodies, or not. I describe fascia as the wrappings of muscles, through muscles, around muscle groups, and through the organs and other tissues of the body—a continuous web work of connectivity that holds us together. Though none of these images conveys the properties of fascia alone, together they begin to give us a fuller picture. We can say, "Fascia is like…" Imagine, for example, peeling an orange, then pulling the pulp out of the individual jackets—fascia is like the jackets, which Ida Rolf called "the organ of support." Image cobwebs going from every part of the body to every other part, à la Louis— connectivity and communication happen, or they don't, if the fascia is blocked. I also imagine our bodies are three-dimensional crocheted body stockings, such that what happens in the big toe may well transmit to the ear. I sometimes suggest that clients and students imagine a piece of cling wrap that's gotten wadded and glued together—fascia will do this unless it remains hydrated. Finally, I suggest tight fascia may make clients feel as if they are wearing five wetsuits, and the third one down is too small and on crooked! These images help clients understand the nature of fascia and its important functions.

Fascia is like…

…the segmented skins of an orange—the organ of support.

…thousands of cobwebs traveling from every part of the body to every other part—a communication network.

…a 3D crocheted body stocking that tugged here will respond there—a transmitter.

…cling wrap that's gotten tangled together and needs hydration—self-gluing in response to stress.

…the body having five or six wetsuits and the middle one is too small and crooked—interfering with alignment and causing pain.

Without confirming this statement with Tom Myers, I assume he also worked with Louis. In his *Anatomy Trains* work[3] he's created myofascial meridian lines of transmission of tension and communication through the body—a system of generic lines he sees in each of us. As I remember Louis' challenge to us all in my class, I suspect Tom was likewise challenged by Louis, spawning his own work, research, and output. And it's good work! It's got more and more therapists thinking about connective tissue, the transmission or lack of it through the fascia, and how we can change the fascial substance for the better by cleaning these lines. Although Tom has proposed that his is a model in progress (and I certainly sympathize with him there; we're never finished!), it's good work he's given us.

Finding that personal line

I prefer my concept of personal lines: **Each client inherently has a combination and culmination of pieces of a variety of meridians and lines that are expressed in him or her alone.** These personal lines are based in part on our activities of daily living, in part on the sum of our experiences that have tried to protect our cores from our environments, and in part on the personality we've developed through our years on the planet. Unlike Myers' lines, they can be superficial *and* deep, or move in changing directions and through different dimensions of the body. Again, they are personal to each of us.

In fact, most of us have a specific personal pattern. Many massage therapists have "kinked" their personal lines from their push off left foot into their hard working right shoulder, and many drivers have contracted both their right psoas and left iliacus and quadratus lumborum, creating left sciatic pain. Many teenage texters have developed "texter's neck" which won't allow their head to fit onto their body. Many computer operators have shoulder and neck issues from their forward posture, with mouse click tension in one hand or the other and carpal tunnel issues in one or both arms.

Various models speak to this idea of congestion with different terms, but somewhere in anyone's personal line is the seed or source of the entire misfortune in the body. We want to find that congestion and get it to relax. We can then ask the rest of that personal line to remain aware, relaxed, breathing, and allow change to happen up and down the entire line as the congestion resolves itself. We need to learn to ask ourselves as practitioners, and challenge client/partners to also search to find: ***Where is the congestion on this personal line, and how do we bring this person awareness of it so they can release that congestion?*** How do we coax them to explore and stretch the primary and secondary congestions on their personal lines, and get these disparate points farther away from each other, while breath moves the entire being and resets the nervous system so they can relax and reboot to the "feel" and "neutral" setting?

As one becomes more familiar with this personal line concept, one also discerns more easily how a client will try to find somewhere else in the body to hide their congestion... If I'm working on someone's psoas muscles, I may see them shorten the back of their neck and put their chin in the air, or clench their fists, or tighten one or both sides of the low back, or turn one or both feet out as they suck up their inner line. If you have a client in standing posture and ask them to bring their head back, you have to monitor not only the head, but shoulders, low back, and even knees as well. It becomes our job to watch more fully the entire being to see where they've tried to hide that pain they say they want to move, but are afraid to release because they're unsure what's on the other side of their known pain. How do we get them to stay in their entire body instead of blocking, holding on, and locking the pain down a bit more tightly?

The environmental slogan "Think global, act local" totally fits this idea. If we can isolate the glitch in the line, then get the client to remain aware both of the stuck spot but also of the rest of the line from top to bottom, keeping that line open through the challenged spot, we'll accomplish much more! Once a practitioner begins to pay attention to the entire personal line of the client as well as the primary congestion (which very well may be the symptom), the client has less opportunities to run away or hide their tension elsewhere until the challenge is released. If one can't hide, one must look at the pattern, and has the opportunity to change it. So, learning to coax the client to stay in the body while part of them wants to run from its blockages is a large part of good movement work as well as bodywork and psychotherapy. And a warning: If you don't receive this work for yourself, you shouldn't be doing it for others! Good therapy is predicated on one having looked at their own issues, first. If you won't explore your own pains and energetic blocks, you'll be less effective with others.

We are how we move

An interesting study is mentioned by Levine in *Trauma and Memory*: Researchers asked convicted non-violent criminals to watch a video of pedestrians walking down a busy street in New York City. Very quickly, these criminals could choose from among the pedestrians whom they would target. For the most part, they made the same choices, which weren't based on race, age, size, or gender...these weren't the important factors that marked people as victims. What researchers found was that several non-verbal signals were present in the "victim": posture, length of stride, pace of walking, and awareness of environment. Those who seemed to walk "on purpose" weren't targeted for crime; those who demonstrated organized movement, flowing motion, "interactional synchrony," and "wholeness"—these people wouldn't be attacked. The researchers posited that criminals could choose people whose walk suggests less self-confidence.[4]

We can enhance our work with clients by simply giving them "homework." However, more appropriately, we might call this homework "homeplay." We can encourage them to focus on one of their patterns that holds them back, or perhaps even two (certainly not three or more!), as we send them back to their world. It may be as simple as remembering to breathe, or drinking more water, or sitting more on the front of their sitting bones at their desk chair, or shifting positions on their long drives. *If we can give them a cue or two* to help them assimilate what we've done in our sessions, we offer them the bonus of both empowering them to do their own healing work and extending the length of the session's effectiveness. Warning: If we give them three or four cues, we've overloaded them and they'll forget them all in their overwhelmed state. I've mentioned mentor Louis Schultz, who used to advise both clients and students, "Now, go home and *play* with this." Good idea to ask for play instead of work, and take the pressure off of the achievers and fighters to come back with correct answers!

Another important distinction: Many who work out seem to be working out with the goal of building strength. If we follow the concept of strength, we realize that too often strength, which is seen as a good thing, can be equated with tightness. Do we really want to add tightness to our bodies? It seems that tightness can lead to brittleness, and something that's brittle is more easily broken or shattered. Therefore, why not forgo strength in favor of its much gentler brother, resilience? I recently experienced just such a client in his bodywork series—a dancer who had overworked and tightened in his workouts, made one lift too many of a dance partner and felt his neck snap, disabling him for over a year before he discovered how to relax the bodymindcore and choose to explore it, soften it, and retrain his body to become resilient instead of strong. It's a strong concept, to be resilient!

And let's also *explore*, along with these cues, the concept of "explore versus achieve." It seems too many clients leave their sessions, go back to their previous world, and immediately try to fit right back into their achievement mode. Often clients ask: "Should I run/work out/do yoga/swim/go back to work today?" My answer is usually something like this: "It depends. Can you go to explore, or will you go to achieve?" If they allow themselves to move right back into achievement mode, they've lost most of the good of the session; yet if they remain in exploration mode, they learn more about themselves, their bodies, and their use of that body in their world. One can overachieve in yoga, swimming, walking, running, or any other form of exploration one might pursue... Can we both encourage this exploration, and demonstrate it to our clients?

So movement work is important! Both learning to watch for movement and its lack, but also helping clients to become aware of their own restrictions and decide to make changes in them, will enhance the effectiveness of our therapies. Conversely, deciding to become the authority for someone, offering them a rote formula in a "one size fits all" type of work, probably won't make one as effective *or* as satisfied with the work one does. Where do you fit?

- One can always be aware that another direction added to a stretch will maximize its effect.

- "Yet movement can be as subtle as slow breathing during sleep."—Louis Schultz[6]

- "I see posture not as how you hold your body when you're still but as how you carry it while you're moving. This distinction reveals posture to be a dynamic activity rather than a static attitude."—Mary Bond[5]

- Each client inherently has a combination and culmination of pieces of a variety of meridians and lines that are expressed in him or her alone.

- I'm interested in getting clients to recognize their personal line with its kinks, glitches, or, perhaps more appropriately, simply congestions...the first step toward release and resolution.

- As one becomes more familiar with this personal line concept, one also discerns more easily how a client will try to find somewhere else in the body to hide their congestion.

- If we can isolate the glitch in the line, then get the client to remain aware both of the stuck spot but also of the rest of the line from top to bottom, keeping that line open through the challenged spot, we'll accomplish much more!

- Why not forgo strength in favor of its much gentler brother, resilience?

- Can you go to explore, or will you go to achieve?

7

Tools and Cues

Fancy equipment isn't essential to help clients find their personal line and its congestions, but it can help anyone's body release that congestion and enhance energy all the way up and down that line. In this book Rob and Liz will use the simplest of tools: mats, bolsters, rollers, balls, etc. It shouldn't take thousands of dollars' worth of equipment to help clients get better! My favorite equipment: my rebounder (the small trampoline for circulation in the legs), balls, and foam rollers; my most expensive piece is a bench that allows me to lie down and extend my body in a way that encourages my six-point star to open and stay open and even hyperextended. None of these bits cost a fortune, and in fact, I think much exercise equipment (some expensive!) used poorly *can be damaging*; including the pieces I've just admitted I use. Too many people have come to me for relief from yoga, weight-lifting, or other workout damage for me to believe otherwise. When I go back to the earlier concept of *exploring* with the equipment instead of believing one must *achieve* with it, the results seem to be much more satisfactory.

As a bodyworker first and movement therapist second, I am "stripped-down"—I don't use many tools or props in my work. I have a few pillows and occasionally will bolster when needed, but my primary tools remain my hands and elbows, my eyes, my words, my assessment, and my empathy. I believe in the "that which we have" school of bodywork, and of cooking.

"That which we have"

Years ago friends were coming for dinner. On looking in the refrigerator and pantry I chose to stir fry vegetables over pasta because those were the ingredients we had at hand. My friend said, "This is delicious! What's it called?" I replied, "That which we have." The next night the same couple returned for dinner again. Without a grocery stop, the second night the same vegetables went into a lentil curry soup. Again, my friend asked what it was called...same answer. I think that which we have is often good enough!

So when I give clients movement cues to explore, I tend to offer ideas or tasks that can be explored in most people's houses or office environments. I believe in using stairs as exercise equipment... likewise, chairs, and counter tops, and doorway trims. Currently my favorite personal "that which we have" is remembering to slow my descent on stairs and remembering to allow my inner arches to slowly reach down and touch the stairs after my toes have connected—as the foot and toes remain truly straight ahead on the stair. All these handy tools, that which we have: I encourage us all to use them more readily. Our ancestors, who worked far harder than we, understood that labor with successful movement was much easier, and it helped them to keep their bodies in excellent condition. So apply "that which we have" to your movement cues. While I can advocate for any and all equipment, I advise you to become a more creative therapist... Find "that which you have," and use it more fully.

Top ten movement cues

1. Remember to breathe!

2. Head up, waist back.

3. Lead with your heart.

4. When walking: If your feet are tires and your knees are headlights, how's your tracking?

5. Can you stay in your toes instead of back on your heels?

6. When standing, stay slightly in front of vertical, on your toes. When sitting, sit slightly in front of your sitting bones, on your toes.

7. Get head, heart, gut, and groin aligned and further apart.

8. Explore all activities while keeping your waist and belly button back.

9. Keep your knees slightly flexed at all times.

10. Explore, don't achieve!

Noah's, Rob's, and Liz's tools

Noah's tools

The tools I normally use in my own day-to-day self work are shown in the illustration below and include:

- foam roller and half roller

- a rebounder/small trampoline

- the bench I use to lay on and practice both flexion and extension

- two pound (0.9 kg) weights

- a stretching strap

- toe spacers, as well as rocking sole shoes and five toe shoes

- various sized balls.

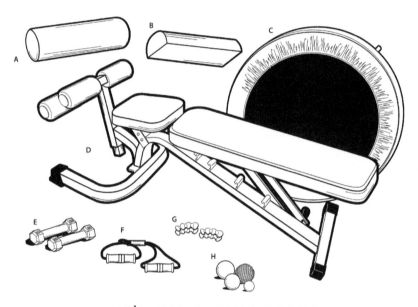

NOAH'S PERSONAL WORKOUT TOOLS:
A) FOAM ROLLER, B) HALF ROLLER, C) REBOUNDER/CIRCULATOR,
D) BENCH, E) TWO POUND WEIGHTS, F) STRETCHING STRAP,
G) TOE SPACERS, H) VARIOUS BALLS.

In Appendix A Rob and Liz offer various techniques to help us help our clients become more proficient and aware in their movement work. I've decided that instead of including a list of equipment needed for any particular protocol, I'll just briefly list what tools each uses in their work. You as therapist can then see their main tools and, in the individual exercises, we will again refer to the tools used.

Rob's tools

Below are all the tools Rob suggests one needs to assist the stretches he'll provide.

- a thin pillow

- a rolled-up towel or head cushions

- a firm and hard ball (i.e., lacrosse, baseball, or hockey ball)

- a firm hardback book or a yoga block

- a medium-sized (approx. 5 inch; 12 cm) inflatable ball

- a firm, small ball (i.e., racquet ball or squash ball).

Liz's tools

Even fewer! They include:

- a chair; sometimes with arms works best, at other times without arms

- a yoga mat

- a 5 inch (12 cm) soft ball

- a blanket, towel, or pillow rolled or folded as needed to use as a prop in various locations

- a theraband or yoga strap.

Words

We've mentioned this fact before in the chapter on communication, but words and mannerisms are great tools in a session! People need to feel cared about, validated, and respected. In order for this to happen, they first must feel heard by you.

Reflective listening suggests one hears a client's complaints, then works to restate their words in such a way that either they can say "Yes, that's exactly what I'm talking about!" or "No, that's not what I mean." If their answer is that they're not feeling heard, it's time to listen more, seek clarification, and work until the minds meet and they feel heard by you. So the first aspect of reflective listening entails just that: listening. Communication needs a message, a hearing of the message by another, the reflection of the message by the second person, and the validation by the first person that the message is received correctly. Most of us are guilty of spending energy deciding what to say next, instead of listening in the present moment. If we can relax and breathe and explore/allow, our clients are more likely to follow, come along, and decide to lead.

A second aspect of good communication is the ability to choose words that are helpful, empowering, and challenging without pushing the client too hard. I've often thought of myself as a cheerleader when I work with clients: "Yes, now, take that right arm a bit longer while keeping that left leg long while breathing...good, there it is! Let that line go!" This choice of words makes sense. So I do consider my words to be among the most important of my tools. (And I'll admit, Rob, I used the word "try" once or twice, because sometimes you just gotta try.)

Many therapists aren't very practiced at talking with clients...but those who can express what they're doing, why, how it will help, and what the client needs to do to be more productive will find their results get better as they learn to use words as tools. This appropriate use of words also leads us right into appropriate assessment.

Assessment

Simple evaluation and assessment allows us to look both at structure for symmetry and balance, but also at the breath or lack of it (my cue to energy flow or its absence), as the keys that help us unlock that person's personal line and its blocks. We simply observe what works and what doesn't in the body, then ask the client for their perspective as to what's going on for them. We add their information to our observations, then formulate a plan to help them unwind that deep stuck personal line, freeing its restrictions. My assessments usually follow that simple formula: I watch a client come in, walk, sit, or stand and I already have ideas about where the problem is anchored in the body and how to help resolve that problem and what needs to happen. Then I look at their intake form and talk with and listen to them describe why they've come. I assimilate their information into my observations and formulate a treatment plan. Then I put them on my table, look again when they're out of the gravity field for yet more info...all before I talk or touch for changes.

Postural assessment and movement assessment are equally useful tools. Imagining a client as having that deep line running through the top of their head, down through their spine, splitting into the adductor compartment, and reaching the ground at the inner arches allows us to look to see where that line has kinks or glitches. Are they balanced foot to foot? Do they put too much weight in the heels, or in one heel? Does one hip live forward or higher, and does one shoulder compensate? Is the head forward, or to one side? These simple observations can tell us much about where the problems reside, but also where they may tend to resolve further up and down the body. Sometimes we can nearly read a client's personal history from their body's patterns.

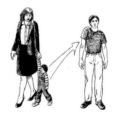 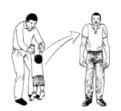 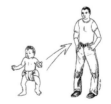

WHAT DO YOU KNOW ABOUT THESE FIGURES? CAN YOU DRAW A CONNECTION BETWEEN EARLY HABITS AND CURRENT PROBLEMS?

Source: From Schultz and Feitis, The Endless Web, *p. 47*

But movement gives us even better clues. Many of us see movement or its lack and pick up our cues as to where we'll want to work on a problem. As a musician, I "hear" the music of the body, of the walk, of the swinging of the arms, of the gait of the hips. Without even needing to walk behind a client to adopt their gait and its glitches, I can often discern just where those glitches reside. Usually when I check in with them, they corroborate what I think I've seen. Other times their information gives me a strong clue as to which pieces of that stuck personal line need work...then, I plan how to honor what they tell me as I also work with what I see.

So, in my work, I first look to see what I see; then I ask the client what they feel. I assimilate those two observations into my treatment plan, work to make the client a partner, and cook with "that which we have." As we work, be it with bodywork, movement work, or even instructing them on how to work for themselves, it's never far from my mind that the more I can get that client aware of these personal line glitches, get them to begin moving into and through their personal restrictions, and keep them breathing, the expensive equipment may be useful, but the simple idea of getting them aware is the most important part of what I offer.

- It shouldn't take thousands of dollars' worth of equipment to help clients get better!

- When I give clients movement cues to explore, I tend to offer ideas or tasks that can be explored in most people's houses or office environments.

- We simply observe what works and what doesn't in the body, then ask the client for their perspective as to what's going on.

The Model of
BodyMindCORE

Echoing Pete Egoscue in *Pain Free*: Good health must begin at the feet and legs and work its way up the body. I agree! Therefore we'll start our examination of my bodymindcore model and its common problems at the feet, then add simple awarenesses/exercises in the appendices to help unwind these problem spots, beginning at the ground and working our way up to the heavens. This chapter focuses on the bodymindcore model; the following appendices present contributions from Rob, Liz, and me: how to release, unwind, and allow energy to flow through each aspect of the body. I'm adding new ideas and information in this book as I find them in my own practice and world. Like Charles Fillmore, co-founder of the Unity movement of religious studies, I reserve the right to change my mind tomorrow! However, the current way I view the bodymindcore follows.

My second book, *Freeing Emotions and Energy (Through Myofascial Release)*, and the third, *Getting Better at Getting People Better*,[1] were both based on my head/heart/gut/groin concept: I see these four as the important landmark centers that need to both move further away from each other and to achieve a straighter alignment as the way to enhance the energy flow through the body. These four landmarks relate to Chinese medicine in that the Chinese see three burners, the groin, gut, and heart, which heat the gut, heart, and head. Superimpose the three burners under the three centers and we find my four centers critical to length, health, and energy flow. These four centers also relate to the four curves of the spine: head = cervical, heart = thoracic, gut = lumbar, and groin = sacral curves. When we focus on lengthening and straightening these four curves, we've further enhanced that energetic flow.

In my world it's this simple: If we can get head, heart, gut, and groin to get further away from each other and also straighter on their line, we've allowed less restriction on that core line I'm chasing and asking clients to identify and relax. I tend to disagree with those who suggest we need more curves in the larger thoracic and lumbar regions, or in the cervical or sacral area. To me, the longer and straighter the spine becomes, the better energy can flow freely from top to bottom and back to top again.

The bodymindcore model can also be compared to and contrasted with the Indian chakra system which has been in use, successfully, for centuries. "Chakra" in Sanskrit means "wheel" and, indeed, usually the seven major chakras are depicted as energetic spinning wheels. They are, from ground up, the survival, sacral, solar plexus, heart, throat, head, and crown. Allowing free and spinning energy through all these seven chakras is the goal of Ayurvedic medicine, and I believe also a worthy goal in any model of health.

For a moment discard the survival or root/ground chakra and the crown or heaven chakra as they're above and below the body (we'll return and retrieve them soon). Once the heart and head have aligned and created space, see the throat chakra as opened too, but also put it aside for a moment. We've now superimposed the chakras onto the head/heart/gut/groin model which is coordinated with the Chinese medicine model. Any model wants space and alignment between these four centers.

Let's envision a new concept in this model by adding five "strictures" or constrictions to the head/heart/gut/groin model: three between these four centers, plus a fourth restriction between the earth or ground and the groin, and a fifth restriction between the heavens and the top of the head. Now our map has five restrictions in addition to our four centers.

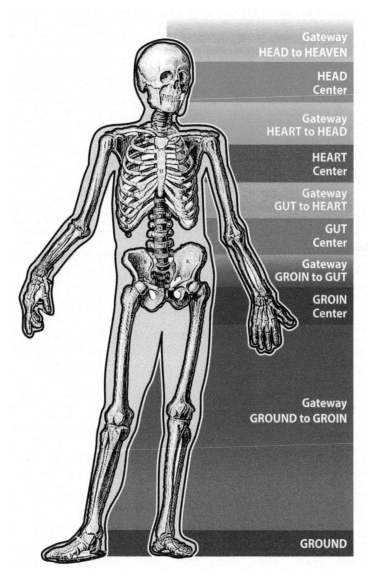

Gateway
HEAD to HEAVEN

HEAD
Center

Gateway
HEART to HEAD

HEART
Center

Gateway
GUT to HEART

GUT
Center

Gateway
GROIN to GUT

GROIN
Center

Gateway
GROUND to GROIN

GROUND

THE BODYMINDCORE MODEL OF CENTERS AND GATEWAYS.

CORE model of gates and centers

Ground to groin **gateway**: the ankles...survival chakra, tib post muscle

Groin **center**: pelvic floor...sacral chakra, pubococcygeal muscles

Groin to gut **gateway**: the rim of the pelvic bowl...no chakra, iliacus, quadratus lumborum and oblique muscles

Gut **center**: the guts...solar plexus chakra...psoas muscle

Gut to heart **gateway**: the primary hourglass...no chakra, diaphragm muscle

Heart **center**: freedom of movement in the ribcage...heart chakra, and intercostal and serratus anterior muscles

Heart to head **gateway**: front of neck and arms...throat chakra, hyoid muscles

Head **center**: cranial diaphragm...third eye/head chakra, scalenes, and upper erector muscles

Head to heaven **gateway**: top of spine...crown chakra, suboccipital muscles

In the past I've used the word "strictures," which means to me a narrowing...something which isn't allowing that energetic flow to move, similar to a clogged hourglass. The word is less important, but the concept is critical. I'm going to co-opt the term *gateways*—similar to, but not the same as, Chinese medicine's gateways. How do we encourage the flow of energy from the ground, through the groin, through the gateway or restriction that separates groin and gut, through the gut, through the separation between gut and heart, through the heart, through the throat restriction into the head, and through the head and on up into the heavens? How do we become a centered bodymindcore being which is able to allow our energetic elevator to stop happily on all nine floors of our body? We'll visit this model more fully soon.

Think of an hourglass; when the sand gets stuck, a light shake or tap can often resume that flow of sand. That's what we're after! If we can simply get clients aware that they're holding energy in a restricted hourglass, and if we can coax breath, energy, and movement through that gateway, we're well on the way to changing the pattern and creating health and energy flow.

We'll feature short comments in this chapter for each of these nine locations on the illustration and work our way up this map, inviting you to consider each of these four centers and five gateways in order from ground to heaven. We'll then invite you to realize: *We can focus attention on opening both the centers and the restrictions between them, through movement cues, touch, and tools, to bring breath and awareness into each of these locations.*

So imagine that between any two centers there's an hourglass that's gotten stuck so sand/energy can't flow through. Between earth and groin we have the pelvic floor muscles acting as that hourglass stricture, which can tighten and stop energetic flow between these earth and groin centers. For me, the ankle hinge is critical to allowing this communication between ground and groin...the ankle is the key to this gateway! Between the groin and gut, we'll focus on the pelvic bowl; the hipbones and their crests and attached muscles restrict flow between centers. Between the gut and heart, the diaphragm muscle and its hiatuses restrict flow from center to center. Between the heart and head, hyoid muscles tighten the throat and stifle creativity as they pull the head down into the heart, which seems to be one of the worst epidemics of our time (text neck!). And between the head and heaven the occiput and sphenoid bones act as a further diaphragm that restricts energy—one could see them as the ceiling of the jaw and the floor of the cranium. So our map now has nine centers and gateways to mind, to observe, and to assess as to where that energetic flow is blocked.

I'm intrigued that Mary Bond in *The New Rules of Posture* suggests six "posture zones": breathing muscles, abdomen, pelvic floor, hands, feet, and head.[2] I find it interesting that four of her zones correlate to mine: breathing muscles = heart, abdomen = gut, pelvic floor = groin, and head = head. The hands and feet are of course tremendously important, and though they may be seen as "sleeve" mechanisms, any thinking person will realize they are also connected to the core. In fact, we can see that, in some ways, Mary supports my six-point star concept—arms, legs, head, and tail—plus the heart and gut, which again I see as core. Whether we look at four, six, or nine spots, we can choose to view the creation of space and movement up and down the line as our primary focus.

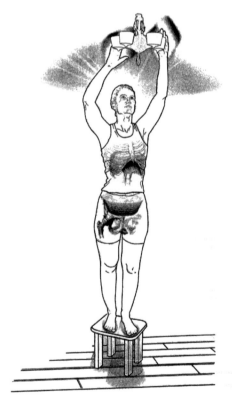

MARY BOND'S POSTURE ZONES FROM *THE NEW RULES OF POSTURE.*

Source: From Bond, The New Rules of Posture, *pp. 9 and 201*

Ground to groin gateway: The ankles

It's important to feel connected to both heaven and earth, but we've got to be grounded. We may have our head in the clouds, but we also need our feet on the ground. We can't be really and fully grounded unless we have supple ankles which give shock absorbency and resilience, a word I use often. So we'll focus on creating awareness of supple ankle hinges as a means to opening the stricture between the earth and the pelvic floor. We can't focus on ankles without their next-door neighbor, the toes; so we'll be including ideas that support ankle flexibility by including toe hinge flexibility and resilience as well.

Simple attention to the way a person walks—where they place their feet, how heavy they are in one or both feet, how flexible the ankles and toes seem to be, or to not be: These are all assessment cues that will tell us whether to ask for more supple ankles. In general, my answer is "Yes!" Look to create more supple ankles and most of the time you'll be rewarded with a more supple body above. As you practice movement cues with clients, and self, let yourself also remember the earlier Rolf quote: "Maturity is the ability to discern finer and finer distinctions." Be more mature in your assessment of any body, including your own.

Notice for yourself: As you stand comfortably, pay attention to your stance. First, does one foot carry more weight? Do toes carry weight, or heels carry more? Or perhaps one toe and the other heel touch the ground more fully; or does the inside of one heel and the outside of the other take more weight? Does one foot turn out more than the other, or the low back feel tighter? Just notice the imbalances, then try to make mild corrections. How strange does it feel to try to find balance between the feet, all the way to the pelvic floor, or even into the low back?

For years I've been monitoring my own body; Rolf's quote above comes back to challenge me as I continue to discern slighter and slighter imbalances between the feet and their translations up through my body, along my personal line. I realize that, as I try to change foot placements and get both feet working together more happily, changes happen above as well. Most of us have a pattern of areas of the plantar surface on one or both feet that don't want to support us physically; if we can get this pattern identified, we can begin to change it. If we won't pay attention and mature in our observations, we won't see change.

Imagine you can ask to remain balanced between the feet while you also place more of the weight in the metatarsal junction between the great toe and the second toe. This point is roughly the "Bubbling Spring" I've mentioned previously—that spot near the front of the foot between big toe and second toe, just in front of the bony junction between the two. It's an important point on the meridian system, and I truly believe well named. If we can walk with a mild spring from this point, much of the problems further up the body will begin to resolve. Experiment with standing and walking from this Bubbling Spring point. After playing with the walk, allow yourself to sink back into your "old" stance and walk. I think you'll feel the difference in the way your body responds to each posture and movement. Can you convey this simple but profound importance to your clients?

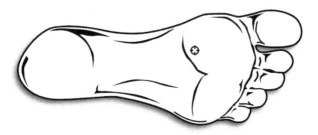

THE BUBBLING SPRING.

Muscles: tibialis posterior (and interosseous membrane), flexors and extensors digitorum and hallucis.

Potential problems: diabetes, cellulitis, knee and foot problems, plantar fasciitis, Morton's neuroma, bunions, high or low arches, varicosities, and edema of the legs all suggest that this person would benefit from the creation of movement and energy through the ankle (and toe) hinge(s). All these problems move farther up into the body as well, but this "grounding" is fundamental!

Groin center: The pelvic floor and pubococcygeal muscles

This center could focus on genitals, though they're below the pelvic floor, and indeed genitals are part of the groin center. But more importantly the tailbone; the sacrum and coccyx are bony parts of a pelvic bowl that includes the pelvic floor muscles...the pubococcygeal (or PC) muscles. We see this center as the sixth point of a body star—the tail. Can it accept energy? Think of these bones as the driver of the entire spine, the spring that creates movement and drives procreation. Can we learn to allow our tail to sag and relax, even if we needn't force it to move? Freeing the sacrum also exercises the pelvic floor and frees the sexual energy often trapped in the groin.

For years I've thought we should all be able to wag our tails! In a perfect world, I don't think we'd be quite so afraid of looking like our co-creatures on the planet who have kept tails...in fact, a statistic I've read indicates that about 1 in 10,000 babies are born with a fairly prominent tail that is cut off surgically at birth. Why shouldn't we have a freely wagging tail? Probably because some million years ago, someone's mother said: "Stop wagging your tail—people will think we're animals!"

Instead of wagging, I think most of us "gird our loins." It's a Biblical injunction: Often, God told his chosen Israelites to "gird their loins" against an upcoming problem or enemy. I believe this concept suggests we tighten our deep line from the ground up; thus, we think of girding loins here.

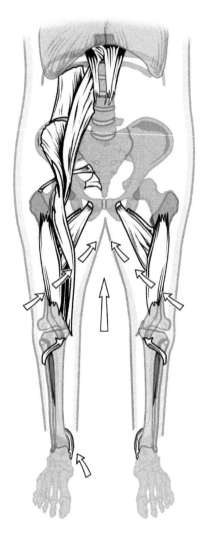

THE "GIRD YOUR LOINS" MUSCLE LINE.

A few cells from the various nervous systems conjoin at the inside front of the coccyx; this area is called ganglion of impar, and isn't even mentioned in many textbooks. It seems these last few cells that integrate all the nervous tissues of the body also relate to this deep, internal, dorsal vagal system that causes us to play dead. When we quit wagging our tail, we lose a useful ability! And we possibly also lose some of our nervous system's integrity...but when we can allow movement in that tail area, we free the pelvis, the bowl, the pelvic floor, the low back, and the sexual organs.

Muscles: pubococcygeal.

Potential problems: sexual dysfunction, bladder issues, endometriosis, difficulties getting pregnant, difficult and painful periods, sacroiliac and sciatic problems, and prostrate difficulties could all be helped by attention to energetic flow in this groin area.

Groin to gut gateway: The pelvic bowl rim and iliac crest

The top of the hip can be seen as the bottom of the stomach. When we work to free hips, we're freeing the groin from the gut. This is a huge stumbling block for many of us; I'd argue, for most of us. Creating freedom in the hips allows energy to move upward into the gut area and then further up the body. For many people, we simply have no energetic flow into the stomach.

The flow of sexual energy is a forbidden topic for too many of us. Some of us were trained by parents who told us to not touch "down there," or by mothers who warned daughters to keep their legs closed at all times. Some experienced early abuse from older people who were expressing sexual energy inappropriately, thus gratifying their needs at the expense of innocent sexual energy. For whichever of many reasons, too many of us have learned to shut down sexual feelings. We won't let the sexual energy—what Wilhelm Reich called the "orgasmic" or orgone energy—rise through the pelvic bowl and into the stomach.[3] If I could give clients permission to find one space and open it, I believe this would certainly rate number one or two on that list. It's critical to allow orgone energy to move upward into the body; yet too many of us keep this gate shut. Reich's attention to moving orgone energy freely through the entire body was curing many health challenges including cancer in the 1940s and 1950s. In part due to his success, his work was outlawed because he used words like "orgasmic" energy.

I've gotten more interested in pushing myself to acknowledge the sexual energy or lack that should arise from this pelvic bowl. To this end, I'll often do stretches in front of a mirror, sometimes in little or no clothing, so I can really focus on seeing, balancing, and accepting the body, but also on bringing the energy into the genitals, up through that pelvic basin, and into the stomach. My concept is this: Make yourself acknowledge the sexual energy that, in too many of us, won't move.

Visualize the pelvis as a bowl: When you carry that bowl, do you carry it in a level fashion, or are you "spilling your guts"? Simply practicing a walk with a level pelvic bowl can realign the body above and below.

I see many people who think they're tremendously overweight, or have a "beer belly." Often, this feeling isn't as true as the fact that their pelvic bowl or basin has tipped forward and they're "spilling their guts" as they hold onto their pelvic floor and tighten the insides of the hips to keep from allowing energy to move through the area. If and when we can stand and walk with a level pelvic bowl and allow energy to move up from the groin, the body responds in a surprising fashion...weight may be lost, sexuality rediscovered, low back pain relieved. Just by opening the stricture between groin and gut—again, one of the most difficult strictures to open—we're inviting not only a whole new spectrum of energy, but also a whole new spectrum of feelings. And remember, pain is resistance to change! Caution: Think back to my earlier three-layer system: layer 1 (what fun and how relaxing!), layer 2 (what's happening to me?), and layer 3 (freezing now). It's easy to push someone into layer 3 if they've not yet discovered this gateway. If you work to help someone open this pelvic area, go gently!

Muscles: iliacus and quadratus lumborum, which I call "ilioquadratus," and obliques.

Potential problems: endometriosis, ibs, digestive issues, incontinence, anxiety, obesity, and/or inability to gain weight.

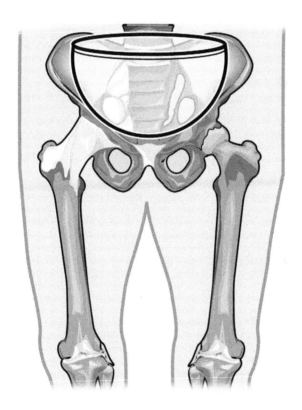

SEE THE PELVIS AS A BOWL WHICH IS
MOST EFFICIENT WHEN LEVEL.

Gut center: The "guts"...solar plexus chakra, psoas muscle

So much should happen in our gut but, as we can't bring energy through that gut/groin gateway, much doesn't get to happen...energy simply can't rise this far in too many cases. This causes so many of our problems above the gut, all the way to the heavens!

I've heard various statistics about the number of people who have endured sexual abuse. I tend to think some of the larger numbers I've seen may be correct, because I believe children are psychically aware and feel some of the abuse that never reaches a physical stage. Between that psychic abuse and the number of people who actually are wrongly treated by someone in power, we learn to shut down in this area too much of the time. How can we bring our awareness back into this painful past, when we're still trying to pretend that painful past hasn't happened? I recall one woman who remembered early sexual abuse just by choosing to slow down, breathe, and focus awareness in her pelvis. When was the last time you visited your own pelvis, and tried to allow energy to rise beyond it, and into your gut? If problems occur below, in the groin, how do we ever get energy to rise past those problems and into the gut? We're disconnected.

I often share a postural image of creating space between a down/ forward genital area and an up/back low back/belly button. Work with this idea; we can all benefit from finding, opening, and toning our psoas muscle, which I feel is key to moving energy into and through the gut.

I've found for myself that one of my simplest and most profound cues is to try to simply remain in activities of daily living with my waistband staying back. Standing, walking, sitting: It's simple, it's not easy. The more that waistband fits back, the more we level our pelvic bowl and the more we allow organs to fit in their assigned spaces more efficiently. I use the image that when standing I prefer to live slightly in my toes as opposed to being in my heels; when sitting, I try to likewise sit slightly on the toes of my sitting bones instead of on the heels...all the while keeping my waist back. As movement therapists, if we can simply encourage attention to this postural detail, we're giving clients a great deal to ponder.

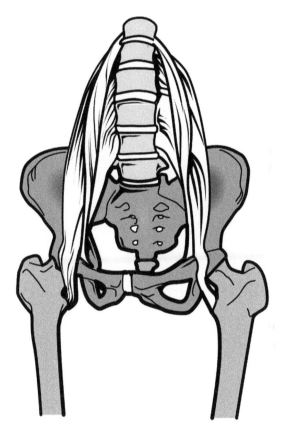

PSOAS, STORER OF ALL STRESS.

And think back to the recent idea of the "beer belly": Those with issues in the stomach area seem to tighten the low back (psoas involvement and flexor withdrawal) and spill their guts. Actually, I believe people who carry additional weight, or even carry weight poorly, are trying to hide, to be invisible! Review the earlier ideas about sexual abuse. Can you see how someone who has been abused would both decide to ignore their groin/gut area, but also put on weight to "hide" and be less attractive?

I've long thought about the words "judgment" and "discernment." I believe the head judges and the gut discerns. For too many of us, especially those who have been challenged early and inappropriately in a sexual realm, it's easier to retreat to the head and live there, judging our world and its inhabitants and events. Can we learn to trust our gut feelings? Often, the gut knows the truth if we can simply listen to it.

Muscles: psoas.

Potential problems: back pain, pancreatic, liver, and gall bladder issues, and ongoing difficulties from long-ago pregnancies, C sections, difficult deliveries, etc.

Gut to heart gateway: The hourglass, the center of it all, diaphragm muscle

My favorite location to make change in a body, and coincidentally, the exact center of this model of five restrictions and four centers! The diaphragm muscle, the muscle of breath, is a main focus of this book. When we can create movement in the area of diaphragm to psoas muscle, we reinstate breath. I see the diaphragm muscle as the ceiling of the stomach and the floor of the heart, and the doorway between them.

For years, one of my most popular courses for bodyworkers has been "The Top Ten Hot Spots to Effect Greater Change." In order, I share my favorite places to work on a body that time after time give good responses and good change. Number one spot in this course: that area below the costal arch where the psoas muscle lands after arising through the inner thighs, up across the pubic region, and anchoring into the front and side of the spinal bones, *as that psoas muscle relates to and nearly articulates with diaphragm cords* which anchor on the front of the spinal bones, very near to the psoas involvement. Simply placing your hands on a costal arch and encouraging breath can have profound results!

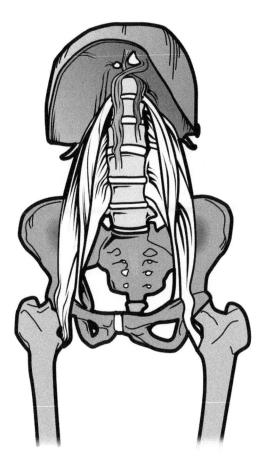

PSOAS FIBERS ASCENDING TO T12, AND
DIAPHRAGM FIBERS DESCENDING TO L2/3.

When I touch a body at this psoas/diaphragm connection, which I also think of as the "heart hinge" or gateway to the heart center, we finally free up a major blockage too many people share. For whichever of many reasons, I believe most of us are holding our breath; a physical, mental, emotional, or energetic trauma has taken our breath away (translate: fighting, fleeing, or playing dead). Until and unless we can get a breath through this major stuck spot, nothing will change in a body. So it behooves us to get better at teaching clients (and ourselves) to find and maintain this full breath. Remember the heart rate variability research: Simply focusing on long and slow breaths contributes to health in more ways than we've yet discovered. And relaxes the fetal curve many of us develop in order to make a smaller target in this unsafe world.

This area is also the psychological storage bin for self-esteem issues; if one feels "less than," this area tends to tighten more. As most of us still go through life with some of that "not good enough" stored in our bodies, one can see how important this spot becomes. Simply getting clients aware of the holding in the sternal area can allow them to begin to release some of their tension, hopefully take that big cleansing breath, and shake out some of their "I'm not good enough" energy from the diaphragm gateway. For me, this is the primary "reboot" I can hope to give a client, either through direct bodywork or through movement and breath cues. Any way we touch and challenge this area can have a powerful impact on the entire body.

I've begun thinking of this important intervention as one form of what I call "vagal reset" and I'm getting more intrigued about both using the technique on nearly everybody who seeks my help, but also teaching more students this simple and effective method for vagal reset. It seems that simply helping clients get a deep in-breath and out-breath, a sort of "shake it out" feeling that courses through the body as a result of release here, can cause them to reorder their lives! This is, happily, a focus of many movement therapies. I hope more of us will consider its importance.

Viewed in another manner, I see this diaphragm muscle as the stricture of the *primary* hourglass of the body—that which separates the upper (head/heart and heavens) from the lower (gut/groin and grounding). If the diaphragm gets tightened (and most are), not only does breath flow poorly, but the energy of the aorta, the esophagus, and the vena cava gets inhibited...energy just can't move appropriately through the body. Learning to get clients breathing into and through this spot can be life changing.

Muscles: diaphragm and psoas.

Potential problems: panic attacks, anxiety, fibromyalgia, chronic fatigue, hiatal hernia, acid reflux, lung issues—all these could be helped by the simple release of this breathing mechanism.

Heart center: Freedom of movement in the ribcage...heart chakra, intercostals, and serratus anterior muscles

The pericardial tissue literally wears out because of lack of circulation; in too many of us it must overwork to accomplish its task. Breath and energy can't reach the heart well enough. By simply moving energy through the diaphragm muscle we allow the heart to work more freely, contributing to enhanced circulation through the entire body. Remember, the diaphragm is the ceiling of the heart; each breath exercises the heart, mildly.

However, perhaps as important as moving the diaphragm itself is the idea of getting the ribs to move with the breath! Many of us grew up singing in choirs where we were taught our shoulders should never move with breath; everything should move from the diaphragm. I disbelieve: To me, everything should move in every direction! When we breathe, our thorax wants to expand laterally, longitudinally, and vertically...we should get wider, deeper, and longer in the thorax. But, in addition, we could allow our ribs to rise and fall similarly to a bucket handle rising from the bucket... the angles or sides of ribs should be able to rise and fall as well. Two muscles seem to stop this rise and fall more than others—the serratus anterior and the intercostals.

Let's look at another issue here: Many of us work to hide our hearts! Whether we were the girl who got breasts, or height, in junior high school before the rest of our classmates; whether we had emotional abusers in our past who caused us to shorten the front of our body; whether we've chosen a job such as computing or driving that encourages us to shorten the front of our body...too many of us tighten this important heart area.

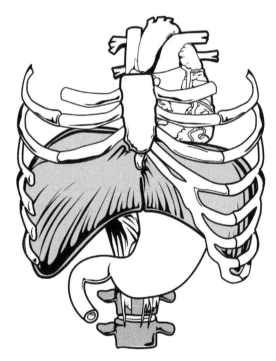

THE HEART IS TRAPPED IN THE RIBS; WHEN THE RIBS
CAN'T MOVE, THE HEART CAN'T WORK FREELY.

I've suggested in the past that clients leave a session "leading with their heart." Some have burst into tears at the suggestion and told me they could never do that! Why not? Why must we hide in our old pain instead of exploring the world that might be? Not only are we hiding our hearts; we're also holding our breath and freezing our ribcages so as to not take up space. How can this be healthy?

I've long thought that, frankly, we're sophisticated roly-poly bugs; when life pokes or prods us, too many of us choose to go fetal. We curl up into that ball (freeze?) and shorten the deep front line, the core, of our body. It's another description of girding the loins. How can we allow that front line to open up so the heart can do its job...especially if our heart isn't in the job we're trying to do? Therefore, living on purpose, meaning loving what you do and doing what you love, contributes to heart health perhaps as much as cardiac health, good diet, and good posture in general.

Muscles: intercostals, serratus anterior.

Potential problems: congestive heart failure, circulatory problems, neckaches, and upper backaches.

Heart to head gateway: The front of the neck and arms...throat chakra, hyoid bone and muscles

Seen as a chakra in the Sanskrit model, the throat opens when the head and heart stay aligned and further apart. When we have a "good head on our shoulders" we're not afraid to express what's in our hearts. In today's neck-forward society, too many of us close this important secondary hourglass. For some, this isn't just about the head/neck-forward problem; it's about the fact that we don't know how to, or are afraid to, express ourselves directly.

Many of us are focused on the old dictums "What will they think? What will they say? If they only knew me, they wouldn't like me." We're afraid to express who we are, what we need, what we'd like our world to be, or not be. We bite our tongue, clench our jaw, and don't "chew them out"—we swallow it. How can we be healthy in the throat area and get the head and heart to talk to each other if we believe we're supposed to live with a shortened, tightened, on-guard throat and neck? And how can we, as movement therapists, encourage movement in and from this gateway?

One of the new diagnoses roaring into our society today is "text neck," a condition in which teenagers are starting to exhibit the arthritic neck conditions of 80 and 90-year-olds. This is critical! We've got to start realizing that, unless we learn to put a head back on our shoulders, we'll be aging far ahead of our time. So simply pulling the head upback and out of the heart is a great first step to opening this gateway between head and heart, and allowing energy through the throat.

For several years I've been hypothesizing that the hyoid muscles, infra- and supra-, are actually the psoas of the neck... As the psoas pulls the spine forward and down and contributes to low back pain, so the hyoid muscles pull the head forward and down toward the body and contribute to neck and shoulder pain.

Make no mistake—if one has a neck problem they have a shoulder problem, and vice versa. So as we work to keep this neck area open, we're also working to remain open in our arms and hands. Rolf instructor Ron McComb stated many years ago, and I quoted in my first book, *Meet Your Body*, that hands are simply an extension of the heart. I agree—while we're thinking primarily of the throat here, I'm suggesting we release arms and shoulders by releasing this throat/neck/heart to head gateway.

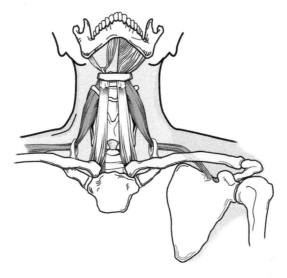

HYOID MUSCLES, THE PSOAS OF THE NECK.

From that perspective, let's think for a minute about arms. When someone presents with problems in their arms and hands, such as tingling, numbness, carpal tunnel, or pain, I'm most interested in finding out what's happening in the lower neck region—c5-7 especially. The nerve supply for the arms erupts from these vertebrae, travels through the front of the shoulder, and is easily impinged, both by the tension we store in our shoulders, and by our lack of movement. Put simply, the more we can open our necks and shoulders, the happier our arms will be.

When I have a client on the table, often their neck is shortened in the back and their chin reaches toward the ceiling. Perhaps they need a pillow behind their head because it won't even reach the table without help. Always, I honor their need for a bolster, but try to wean them away from the idea that they need to use something to support such a terrible posture. Some people in a standing posture can't get their head back anywhere close to where it belongs on the top of their body. If we can't get that head to fit upback, horizontal or vertical, how can we ever get the client to have a "good head on their shoulders"?

Muscles: infra and suprahyoids, pterygoids.

Potential problems: temporomandibular joint (TMJ), dental issues, neck and shoulder problems, carpal tunnel, thoracic outlet syndrome, vertigo, psychological illnesses.

Head center: Flushing the brain... third eye/head chakra, scalenes, and upper erector muscles

The head pulled down and forward by the closed throat/neck/shoulders causes a fogginess of the brain; the lack of circulation means energy can't reach the brain. Once we can open that throat channel (usually, the diaphragm needs to be opened first) and allow energy to reach the head, amazing things can happen! People can think and reason clearly; headaches often disappear; life is more fun. And as we've said, too much of life is lived in this head-forward position; how can we possibly feed energy to a head that can't fit on top of a body?

Louis Schultz says:

> Many people have a tendency to carry their heads as though they were independent structures. A more workable image is to consider the skull as a great big vertebra sitting on top of the spine. This allows us to visualize how the head can move "in line" with the rest of the spine. When the movement of the spine is like a spring, the head is its last segment.[4]

I like both the concept of the head as the final vertebra, but also the spine as a spring! We all could become a bit more bobble-headed to feel healthier. I like to imagine I can simply lift my head upback, lengthen the back of my neck, and invite my chin to travel straight back, thereby restoring my head back onto my body.

How can we ever find energy through the entire line if we can't get energy through our necks and into our head? How can we attune to Universal Energy if that occiput is jammed into the neck? We've got to create length between occiput/c1/c2, what I think of as an "atlas wedge" where c1 has migrated forward and is being pinched by occiput and c2, causing a constricted spinal column, a mind fog, a headache, and a general disorientation.

Ida Rolf located a bundle of nerves near what could be called the "third eye" in a few anatomy textbooks; this bundle is called "ganglion of rebes." If we remember the negative junction box that I believe the ganglion of impar forms at the base of the spine, does it make sense that its counterpart should be at the top of the spinal cord? For me it's totally possible that these two ganglia form the top and bottom of the entire nervous and electrical system of the body. Do you see yet another reason we'd like to get breath, movement, alignment, and energy from the base ganglion to the top one?

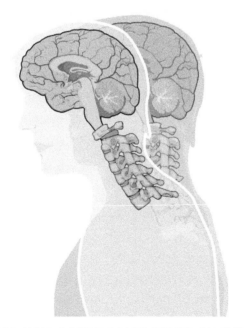

A FORWARD HEAD POSTURE PUTS STRESS ON THE ENTIRE
SPINE AND CAUSES MANY OF OUR PROBLEMS.

Muscles: hyoids and upper erectors.

Potential problems: senility, forgetfulness, stroke, carotid blockage (see this as another entry to vagal reset as the vagus descends through the carotid channel in the side of the neck).

Head to heaven gateway: Head in the clouds...crown chakra, occiput, and sphenoid bones

When the occiput, atlas, and axis get congested, partly due again to a head-forward posture, but also to unprocessed thought forms, a tension arises in the back of the neck as it meets the skull. How can we be part of something larger, of the universe, when we can't find and maintain our connection to some sort of "higher power"? When the bones in the center and back of our head get jammed, we can't think, we can't reason, and we can't function in the world as well as we'd like.

One of my mentors used to use the language of demons and entities in relation to this tension in the back of the neck; I chose to revise the language to "unprocessed thought forms." Whether one thinks in terms of demons or not, *something*, some thought, chooses to reside in this area when we allow it to do so. Often that thought is as simple as "I'm not good enough, I don't do enough. I must work harder and achieve more to get ahead." Perhaps even more often these days, that thought is "I'm not sure I'm safe here and now." If we pay attention and remove these thought forms regularly, we can keep a good head on our shoulders.

I often talk to clients, and students, of the idea that the general is the fellow who sits or stands on top of the hill and watches the overall picture of the battle or the war. He doesn't usually get into any danger himself; he's on top watching the unfoldment of the entire picture. The foot soldier, on the other hand, is on the front line, sticking his neck out, and is likely to get his head blown off. Which are you? Which clients do you see as foot soldiers in their own battle with life?

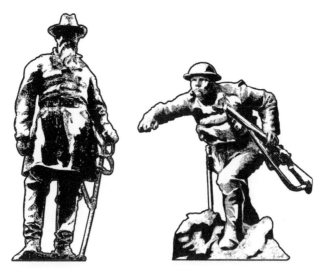

THE GENERAL? OR THE FOOT SOLDIER? WHICH ARE YOU?

Let's also consider that the bones in the cranium are meant to be moveable…too many seem to forget this fact. Yet, craniosacral therapists understand the virtue of keeping the sutures, or joints, of these bones moveable if we're to maintain health in the head and cranium. Simply believing movement in this cranium is possible opens us to explore a healthier head and neck.

Muscles: suboccipitals.

Potential problems: fogginess, migraines, strokes, and mental illnesses.

Conclusions

So, what began as the realization that I'd like to get everyone on the planet to open their heart hinge has progressed to the certainty that I'd like to teach us all to more fully align and lengthen the groin, gut, heart, and head centers, thus opening the four main curves of the spine. To this work I've now added the idea that, to be fully alive, we need to open all gateways from the ground to the heavens and teach our body's elevator to stop at all nine floors.

These are the centers and gateways of the body which movement therapists (and others) can focus on retraining, releasing, moving energy through, getting breath to open, and creating health in them. Rob and Liz created the first appendix to this book which gives specific techniques and tools to work with each space, to create the flow of health from the ground to the heavens, through the gut/ groin/heart/head centers and their respective restrictions. Of course we realize this model won't necessarily serve every person in every situation, but I believe it serves well much or most of the time, and I think their specific exercises can free these restrictions. How do we create space and resilience in all centers and gateways, allowing energy and breath and circulation to flow through the entire being, and feel the free movement of both the core of this body and its six points as we travel up and down the elevator?

So, most of my work is done! As I conclude my main contribution to the book, I'd like to recap a few conclusions. I'd suggest holding onto these ideas: First, *any* therapy can be helpful, if the client can see the value, feel safe, and decide to participate. As you can see from my words, I believe movement, breath, and exploration to be the critical factors when making changes in a body—and the deeper we want to go, the slower we must drive! I've realized in my own body that the deeper I want to go in looking at restrictions, the slower I *must* go. Slow and deep exploration lets me change. And last, consider your partnership with clients to be something of a semi-tough-love parenting; it's important to push clients to explore without pushing them into resistance. It's best if you can convince them to work alone, preferably with a mirror to observe where they hide and where they overwork. If you become their expert, you've deprived them of the opportunity to be master of their own process.

I've given my model, my ideas, my philosophy of bodymindcore, the work we can do to enhance that core experience, and why we want to do it. The appendices are primarily for Rob and Liz, though I'll add thoughts in all as well. (All three of us contribute to the appendices, so the headings are color-coded according to who wrote each section—Noah's headings are blue, Rob's are green, and Liz's are orange.) I invite you to use the appendix ideas as guidelines and references...turn to their exercises when you suspect specific blocks in individuals who come to you for help. We can change people's lives by getting them to move with awareness, energy, and breath. It's important work we have... Good luck, on your personal journey, and on the journey with your clients.

- We have nine centers and restrictions to mind, to observe, and to assess as to where that energetic flow is blocked.

- Look to create more supple ankles and most of the time you will be rewarded with a more supple body above.

- Freeing the sacrum also exercises the pelvic floor and frees the sexual energy often trapped in the groin.

- Creating freedom in the hips allows energy to move upward into the gut area and then further up the body.

- I've found for myself that one of my simplest and most profound cues is to try to simply remain in activities of daily living with my waistband staying back!

- I see the diaphragm muscle as the ceiling of the stomach and the floor of the heart, and the doorway between them.

- When we touch a body at this psoas/diaphragm connection, which I also think of as the "heart hinge" or gateway to the heart center, we finally free up a major blockage that many people share.

- The throat opens when the head and heart stay aligned and further apart.

- When the movement of the spine is like a spring, the head is its last segment.

- When the bones in the center and back of our head get jammed, we can't think, we can't reason, and we can't function in the world as well as we'd like.

Appendix A

Gateway and Center
Self-Release Series

Our three appendices are designed to give exercises and awarenesses that many movement therapists might not have yet considered, and are based on the idea of opening specific centers and gateways of the body. As in the previous chapter, we'll begin at the ground and work our way up the body. In Appendix B we'll focus on more subtle work, trying to pull that rubber band in more directions—thus asking various centers and gateways to pull further from each other. Though some of that subtle work will appear in this appendix, Appendix B will encourage you to "Make it up!" Each section here in A will feature thoughts from Noah (blue headings) about opening restrictions on the targeted center or gateway, followed by illustrated cues from Rob (green headings) or Liz (orange headings). I've also added a short Appendix C called "Maturity." I hope one finds long-term challenges in it. For now, here are Rob and Liz.

Introduction

I first discovered Noah and his bodymindcore approach in 2007 while searching for more answers on the formidable psoas muscle. I enrolled on his weekend workshop hoping to be educated on this vital piece of anatomy and, instead, I was blown away! Noah's "Psoas: Storer of All Stress" workshop not only made clear how the psoas could be the cause of several physical ailments, but it also taught me to consider that the psoas could be harboring emotional trauma as well. In fact, the benefits of learning more about the psoas through Noah's approach were "eye-opening" enough that I immediately signed up to his bodymindcore series to learn more!

I've always appreciated that my physical therapy degree could only provide me with the required foundational skills to diagnose and treat my clients, and that, in order to become a better and more effective practitioner, I would need to undertake further education. The first significant step I made to improve clinical effectiveness was deciding to pursue a better understanding of human movement (biomechanics). Following the advice of a great mentor and colleague, I chose to begin practicing the original Pilates method. It was soon apparent how this movement therapy approach would complement the manual therapy work I already offered, so a year later I studied Pilates with one of the world's leading authorities. My Pilates training consolidated the importance of studying my clients' movement—observing, feeling, and listening to how they used their bodies—and also taught me to help them move better, reduce reoccurrence of injury, and optimize their task performance.

Meeting Noah a few years after my Pilates training, and working with his approach, immediately drew parallels with the manual therapy skills gained from my physical therapy degree and the movement therapy in the Pilates method. Noah and I very quickly began to share techniques for optimizing our clients' experience, sharing the common goals of coaxing release, restoring energy, and educating on better movement practice.

This book is the result of several years of Noah and I exploring the thoughts and experiences of physical and emotional trauma witnessed in our day-to-day practice. I've always believed Noah's work would be of benefit to any movement therapist despite his training being geared more often to the manual therapist.

My intention with the series of exercise "examples" is to help you, the movement therapist, begin to understand how this approach can be applied to your work. I hope they illustrate how you too can begin to coax your clients to release physical and emotional trauma further, moving past the "sticky" strictures or restrictions, freeing up the *flow* of energy, and ultimately restoring breath and movement to clients.

The examples that follow are simply that—examples! As Noah would profess in his training, we intend to give you, as a chef, the ingredients to work with, rather than provide a cookbook with a recipe to follow.

I've found these exercises relating to respective gateways and centers will help the client achieve better flow through their bodies; but they're by no means an exhaustive list. I strongly encourage you to build from my ideas as well as Liz's and Noah's, apply the bodymindcore principles to your own method, and witness the amazing results they can achieve!

In my attempts to convert bodymindcore manual work into self-release prescriptive exercises, I found myself employing the use of several props. As a movement therapist I'm sure you're familiar with the items described within the text, but again, don't be afraid to utilize something else that you feel achieves the same result. Often our clients may not have access to these pieces of equipment, so part of your challenge is to discover what else would suffice (Noah's "that which we have").

I start the self-release series with four simple "check-in" exercises which I've found provide both me and my clients with a good objective and subjective measure of the effectiveness of gateway and center exercises. Returning to these positions after trying some or all of the exercises should elicit significant positive feedback.

I sincerely hope you enjoy!

Check-in process

Positions 1–4

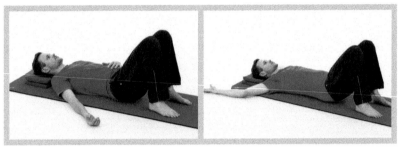

Position 1 Position 2

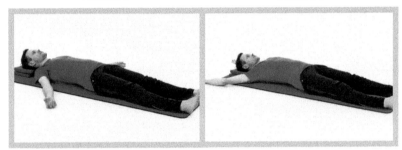

Position 3 Position 4

STARTING POSITION

Lie semi-supine with knees bent and feet flat, hip width apart, with pressure balanced between heels and toes. Arms are relaxed and open out to the side with palms facing the ceiling to allow shoulders to widen. Head rests on supportive pillow, allowing neck to remain long both front and back.

EXERCISE: POSITION 1

- Breathe in "slow and low," aiming to fill the abdominal cavity between the top of the pelvis and base of the ribcage.

- Trickle the air in to allow time to send it throughout the abdominal region (front, back, and both sides).

- As the abdominal cavity fills, feel for the abdomen slowly rising toward the ceiling.

- At the top of your inhalation, pause for a few seconds and think and feel for areas of tension in the body.

- Begin a slow exhalation, targeting the areas that felt tight and restrictive to the breath.

- Use the full exhalation to make the body feel heavier on the floor, from the tip of your toes to the top of your head.

EMPHASIS

- Achieve heaviness in the entire body, feeling for the contact with the floor along the length of the spine.

- Try not to tense in the body and focus on letting the arms and legs release from the center.

- Breathe in through pursed lips—like sucking from a straw—allowing more time to direct the breath where necessary.

IMAGERY

- Visualize the body laid out on sand and consider the indentation it leaves—make it deeper with each breath.

- Use your breath to allow the body's weight to release heavier into the sand.

AVOID

- using your normal breath pattern and inhaling too quickly.

- holding tension in the shoulders and neck as you breathe—aim for the abdominal region.

REPETITION

- At least four "slow and low" breaths.

MODIFICATION

- If lying on your back is uncomfortable, try the same principles sitting tall on a chair.

Continue with the same breathing as above, but begin to lengthen and challenge your body:

- **Position 2**—Lengthen both *arms* above the head as best as possible—let them become heavy.

- **Position 3**—Lengthen both *legs* away from the pelvis—let them become heavy.

- **Position 4**—Lengthen *arms* and *legs* away from the trunk—let them *all* become heavy.

Here we begin examples to help you help your clients find their core experience in each specific gateway and center more fully. In each segment, we'll first visit Noah's more philosophical ideas—you'll have to work a bit to explore his thoughts! Next Rob, then Liz, will add their favorite ways to challenge clients to more fully find core. Please see this section as a reference work and not a protocol...find the exercises you think can best help the individual client!

Ground to groin gateway

I've long been a fan of "big toe pushups," whereby I simply stand as balanced as possible, then ask my big toes to lift my body straight up, *and* down, *slowly*. It's amazing how often my outside toes want to take on the task instead; it's really a struggle to keep that energy rising, and falling, through the big toe hinges. Can you see and feel how this big toe pushup work asks ankles to become more resilient as well? Perhaps most important is the slow motion working of the plantar arch surface: As we create awareness and resilience in the space between heels and toes, we develop a healthier personal line. This isn't a portion of our body we spend time and energy finding and exercising, to our detriment.

For an added challenge, try mild knee bends, which encourage ankle function. Then from a mildly bent knee position, begin the big toe pushups again. Experiment/explore...find the pieces of toe hinge and ankle hinge that don't want to support or work for you, in one or both feet, and ask for awareness and change in that unused and unexplored place. Use your arms to help if necessary—even holding onto a counter, chair, or railing if you need support or arm strength to maintain balance. Challenge the toes, ankles, and knees to participate in your movement. To challenge self even more, work to slow down the rise and fall of your body, calling on smaller and smaller muscular motions.

Those cultures who spend time in a squatting position have far less back and bowel problems than our own culture in the Western world, as well as healthier ankles. It seems we'd all be served by learning to squat more of the time. Occasionally I'll start a course by asking students to squat for 10 or 15 minutes. Most of us can't do it!

I'm a fan of the small trampoline usually called a circulator or rebounder; it's perhaps three feet (1 m) across and six inches (15 cm) off the ground. This small and gentle trampoline takes much of the shock out of both toe pushups and knee bends, and assists the ankles in allowing squatting as well. Simply using a rebounder slowly for 10 or 15 minutes at a time encourages toe and ankle hinge movement as well as massaging the entire core line through the pelvic floor as it sends an energetic flow all the way to the crown. Warning: The first time I stepped on my rebounder after my wreck, I could only achieve three toe lifts before wearing out! Don't push too hard.

Let's put awareness of walking into the equation. You've witnessed many interesting and varied gaits in your practice, and out on the street. Too many of us are too heavy in our heels, or shuffle our feet, or nearly tiptoe through life. The use of a full ankle hinge, toe hinge, and the arches that should be exercising in between them just doesn't happen often enough. We need to push off from the ground with our toes, transmitting energy to the ankle. No toe hinge? No ankle hinge either. As that movement begins and the ankle opens, the knee opens, the hip opens, and on up the line. If nothing moves below, nothing moves above.

But if we can find that space between toes and ankles, ask it to stretch, to lengthen, to open: We've opened the entire body. This midfoot area is critical—it's your connection to the earth. Poor articulation in this midfoot means we don't allow weight to transfer between heel and toe, limiting our ability to absorb the shocks of our steps, and impacting the entire body above the feet as we protect arches and ankles. If the sole of each foot has more than 7000 nerve endings that work together, can you see how not using the feet is yet another way to suck our inner line up, to gird our loins, and to not allow ourselves to live on a safe planet?

CUES

Image: Create matching feet and legs.

Simple: Attention to walking; big toe pushups.

Complex: Mild knee bends with toe pushups, in slow motion. Squatting.

Assisted Rolling the Sole Release

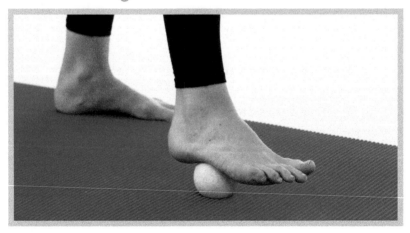

STARTING POSITION

Stand tall, lengthening up through the spine. Place sole of one foot on top of a firm, hard ball (lacrosse ball, baseball, or hockey ball).

EXERCISE

- Apply progressively firmer pressure onto the ball and roll the ball along the length of the sole.
- Travel from the ball of the foot all the way to the heel.
- As you apply pressure, think and feel for any restriction along the way.
- Stay at the restriction and inhale "slow and low"—aiming to reach and release the tension.
- Pause at the top of the inhalation and focus on the tension and congestion.
- Use the full exhalation to make the tension soften and the breath to pass through it.

EMPHASIS

- Feel heaviness in the sole of foot and widening foot contact with the floor.
- Release the tension to increase the *flow of breath*.
- Work more on the foot that talks the loudest!

IMAGERY

- Visualize the foot melting over the ball and becoming as wide and soft as it can become.

AVOID

- applying *too much* pressure: increased pain = increased tension.

- bending at the waist to apply the pressure—stay tall and keep the other gateways as open as possible.

REPETITION

- At least four "slow and low" breaths.

MODIFICATION

- If standing while rolling makes you too sore, try the same movements sitting up tall in a chair.

PROGRESSION

- Lengthen along the Line—with improved balance, work toward reaching high to the ceiling with an arm/arms.

Assisted Tibialis Posterior Release

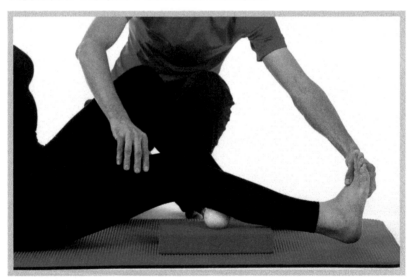

STARTING POSITION

Sitting up tall, supported by the hands placed behind back, drape one leg over a firm, hard ball on a yoga block or even a hardback book, so the ball applies pressure to the center of the calf muscle, just below knee joint. Bend other knee and place foot flat on the floor to offer more support.

EXERCISE

- Apply progressively firmer pressure onto the ball, rolling the ball along the length of the calf area.

- Travel from the back of the knee all the way to the top of the Achilles tendon.

- As you apply pressure, think and feel for any restrictions along the way.

- Stay with the tension and inhale "slow and low"—aiming to reach the restriction with breath.

- Pause at the top of the inhalation and focus on the restriction.

- Use the full exhalation to make the tension soften and the breath to pass through it.

EMPHASIS

- Feel heaviness throughout lower leg and in sole of the foot.

- Release the tension to increase the *flow of breath.*

- Aim to create heaviness in ankle.

IMAGERY

- Visualize lower leg as a piece of rolled-up dough: As you roll the leg over the ball, think of the dough being rolled out flat.

AVOID

- applying *too much* pressure: increased pain = increased tension.

REPETITION

- At least four "slow and low" breaths.

- If sitting tall is uncomfortable, consider resting your back against the foot of a sofa or wall.

PROGRESSION

- Feel for any restriction, then pull that tension from the *end* of the line—flexing and extending toes.

Tapping Toes

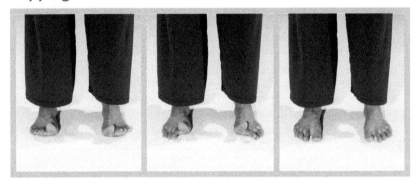

STARTING POSITION

Find a relaxed stance with spine tall, back of waist and back of neck back, with feet about shoulder width, and knees soft and rooted into the ground.

EXERCISE

- Energy goes where breath goes. Movement goes where energy and breath go. Connect the breath into the soles and toes as each toe touches the floor.

- Lift all toes up, while keeping the rest of the feet on the floor.

- Lower one toe at a time, beginning with pinky toe.

- When you have reached big toe, repeat again.

EMPHASIS

- Keep the rest of the body relaxed.

- Feet stay grounded on the floor and only toes move.

- Play with the idea of breathing into the toes and soles of your feet, all the way to the top of your head.

IMAGERY

- *Imagine* tapping your toes one by one to the beat of light music, while the rest of the foot stays down.

AVOID

- using any other muscles in your torso to create the movement, such as head forward or tensed shoulders.

REPETITION

- As many times as you like.

MODIFICATION

- If unable to stand, sit on a chair, spine tall, legs parallel to the floor, knees at 90 degrees, and feet grounded on the floor. Avoid slouching in this position.

- Do one foot at a time.

PROGRESSION

- Reverse the movement, by tapping the toes from big toe to little toe.

Pulling the Towel

- Place a towel underneath your feet. Lift and stretch your toes on the towel as far they can reach.

- Use your toes to pull the towel toward your heels.

- Only the heels stay firm and grounded.

- Progress by pushing the towel away after pulling it toward your heels.

Ankle Flexion and Rotation

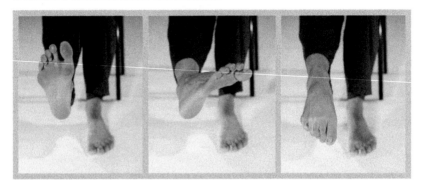

STARTING POSITION

Sit on a chair, pillow, or floor, whichever is comfortable enough to sit upright without creating tension or cramping in the hip flexors. If seated, feet are grounded, knees are at a 90 degree flexion, and hamstrings are parallel to the floor. Spine is elongated while shoulders are relaxed; then extend one knee only high enough so that the foot can move freely. Try having your hips slightly more anteriorly tilted.

EXERCISE

- Inhale into toes, spreading them away from each other. Exhale; squeeze toes together.

- Inhale; turn both feet to right. Exhale; return to center. Back and forth.

- Inhale into soles of the feet, and lift one inner arch and the other outer arch. Exhale; return soles to the floor. Lift and return opposite arches in same way, with breath.

- Inhale into heels; plantarflex. Exhale; dorsiflex.

- Draw circles, infinity symbols, and other shapes with your toes and foot.

EMPHASIS

- *Only* feet and toes move.

- Maintain a light and lifted spine with conscious, mindful movements. Be creative! Move them how you like!

IMAGERY

- Imagine your feet slow dancing to your favorite ballad and no one else is watching.

AVOID

- overtensing shoulder.

- allowing head to creep forward.

- locking elbows and gripping the chair too tightly.

REPETITION

- As needed, as preferred.

MODIFICATION

- Slow the movement down.

- Keep foot on the floor while still opening/closing/moving.

PROGRESSION

- Add a theraband or yoga strap under arches or on the floor to press and release and create shapes with added resistance.

Groin center

Simply lie on your back—floor, bed, wherever you can become comfortable. Then focus on breathing to your tailbone. Now, imagine you can wag your tail, without moving anything! I've actually had several people over the years who could truly wag their tails from side to side. I think it's less important to be able to really wag, and more important to believe it would be all right for the tail to get loose and wag, as the pelvic floor relaxes. So while I don't encourage anyone to *achieve* a freely wagging tail, I encourage them to explore that feeling.

Perhaps by pulling one leg long while jamming the other straight leg up into the tailbone (while breathing and exploring), one can both feel the sacroiliac junctions more fully, but also begin to find this tail that, for too many of us, has been tucked between our legs like a whipped puppy dog. Wag it! Create movement and resilience in the tailbone area. Many clients have told me they manage their own sciatic problems with this simple movement. Be sure to change legs as well.

While on the floor or bed, and focusing on the breath to the tailbone, also allow yourself to find and feel your genital area. Many of us are simply afraid to let energy reach the genitals! Allow yourself to breathe into and experience movement in the genital area as well as the tailbone, and allow sexual feelings, if they should arise, without judgment.

Over the past 40 years, we've been given the "Kegel" exercise, named for a doctor who realized women with incontinence issues, particularly after pregnancy, could enhance the tone of their pelvic floor simply by starting and stopping the flow of urine during the urination process. For years, this exercise has helped incontinent women and men. In the past several years, a new problem has emerged: Some younger women who have been hypertoning their PC muscles with this exercise are developing too-tight pelvic floors and are actually *creating* incontinence! So while Kegel exercises still seem a viable way to enhance urinary continence, it seems like, as with so many other ideas, one can overdo in the need to achieve instead of allowing exploration.

Remember the "gird your loins" line from the tibialis posterior; adding in the adductor, psoas, diaphragm, and above? If we can create awareness in the adductor compartment, we're opening this pelvic floor. Ida Rolf was a believer in finding pelvic integrity; she felt it was key to any being learning to live happily on the planet. She encouraged us to learn to sit (her least favorite body posture) more healthfully by sitting slightly forward of our sitting bones, allowing the pelvis to rock, and letting the pubic bone drop slightly toward the chair and elevating the tailbone. That movement gives a spring-like action. I often suggest clients stand, then rock *slightly* back and forth (front to back) until they are just slightly in the toes. I encourage the same idea with sitting bones as well. Can we sit slightly in the toes of our sitting bones instead of in the heels? Can we ungird our loins in the feet and legs and the pelvic floor as well?

CUES

Image: Be the Pink Panther, with a long and heavy tail that only wags clear down at the floor.

Simple: Lie down and pull one leg long while jamming the other into the sacrum; then reverse. Breathe!

Complex: Adductor stretches, preferably on back with legs up the wall, heels on the wall, and allowing feet and legs to simply spread toward the floor.

Assisted Inner Thigh Release

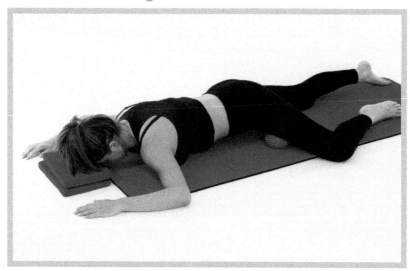

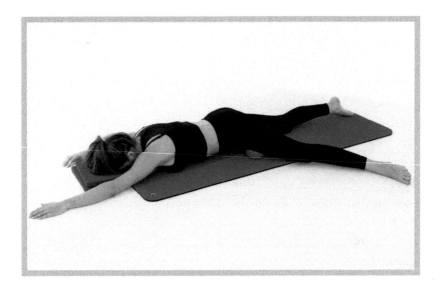

STARTING POSITION

Lie prone. Rest your forehead on a pillow so neck is long front and back and nose is clear of the floor. Abduct a leg out to the side, bringing knee up high and resting inner thigh on top of an inflatable 5 inch (12 cm) ball. Start with the ball up close to the origin of adductor, as near to pubic bone as possible.

EXERCISE

- Apply progressively firmer pressure onto the ball and roll the ball along the length of the inner thigh.

- Travel from near pubic bone out toward inside of the knee joint.

- As you apply pressure, think and feel for any restrictions along the way.

- Stay at the tension and inhale "slow and low"—aiming to reach the stricture.

- Pause at the top of the inhalation and focus on releasing the tension.

- Use the full exhalation to make the restriction soften and the breath to pass through.

EMPHASIS

- Feel heaviness throughout thigh and down leg.

- Release the tension to increase the *flow of breath*.

- Relax into the posture and keep the body heavy to the floor.

IMAGERY

- Visualize thigh like a plastic bottle of water: As you roll leg over the ball, think of the plastic bottle changing shape as the water moves around.

AVOID

- applying *too much* pressure: increased tension = increased pain.

- creating tension higher up in the shoulders.

REPETITION

- At least four "slow and low" breaths.

MODIFICATION

- If the ball is too uncomfortable, consider using a rolled-up towel over a broader surface area.

PROGRESSION

- When you find a restriction, then straighten the knee and lengthen the arm.

Self Inner Thigh Release

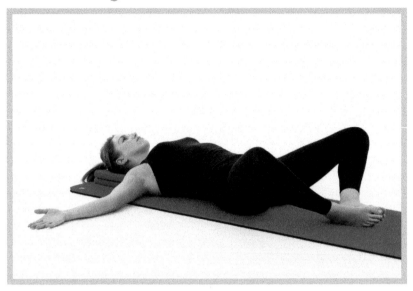

STARTING POSITION

Lie semi-supine with knees bent, relaxed out wide, and soles of feet together. Arms are relaxed and open out to the side with palms facing the ceiling to allow the shoulders to widen. Head rests on supportive pillow, allowing neck to remain long both front and back.

EXERCISE

- Breathe in "slow and low," aiming to fill abdominal cavity between the top of pelvis and the base of ribcage.

- Trickle the air in to allow time to send it throughout abdominal region and into groin.

- As the air travels further, think and feel for the restrictions in the inner thigh.

- At the top of your inhalation, pause for a few seconds and try to think and feel for areas of tension in thighs.

- Begin a slow exhalation, targeting the areas that felt tight and restrictive to the breath, asking them to relax.

- Use the full exhalation to make sacrum feel heavier on the floor and inner thighs longer.

EMPHASIS

- Feel heaviness throughout thigh up to sacrum.

- Release the tension to increase the *flow of breath*.

- Relax into the posture and keep the body heavy to the floor, including shoulders.

IMAGERY

- Visualize inner thigh like a wooden pole coming from pubic bone out to knee. As you exhale, see the wooden pole change into a piece of pliable elastic that lengthens under load.

AVOID

- quickly dropping knees out wide.

- forcing the soles of feet together—allow them to move as required.

REPETITION

- At least four "slow and low" breaths.

MODIFICATION

- If the position is too uncomfortable, consider bolstering knees with something on either side (cushions, pillows).

PROGRESSION

- Consider lengthening the line further by reaching arms higher above the head.

Pelvic Rock

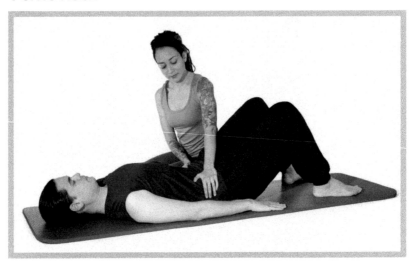

STARTING POSITION

Supine, soft, and lengthened on the floor. Knees bent and hip width apart (add soft ball or pillow to stabilize knees if necessary); feet aligned with the knees; heels 2–3 inches (5–8 cm) away from the sitting bones. Pelvis and spine are in a neutral position. *If assisting, kneel beside client and place your hands on both sides of their hips.*

EXERCISE

- Inhale into the front of the body to anteriorly tilt or arch hips, lifting lumbar spine, and allowing tailbone to lightly touch the floor, creating a small space under lumbars.

- Exhale from back of body to posteriorly tilt hips, allowing tailbone to lift slightly and imprint spine.

EMPHASIS

- Practice mindful rocking of pelvic floor from anterior to posterior tilt.

- Return spine to relaxed position on the floor.

- Allow a slight chin nod toward chest, with back of neck remaining long.

- Keep knees and feet aligned with anterior superior iliac spine (ASIS) and parallel to each other.

IMAGERY

- Draw a vertical line, up and down, with your tailbone.

- Visualize balancing a bowl of water on your hips; arch and imprint hips to tilt the bowl.

AVOID

- overexaggerating anterior tilt, causing lumbar/sacral discomfort.

- overexaggerating posterior tilt, jamming lumbars into the ground.

- lifting chin and extending the back of the neck.

- tensing shoulders.

REPETITION

- As needed, as preferred.

MODIFICATION

- Place a small folded towel under occiput to maintain chin nod and neck length.

- Place a small twisted towel under lumbars to help keep the spine in line as well as aid in teaching hips and spine to feel lumbar space in an arch. When the client rolls the spine up into the Pelvic Rock, he or she will be able to feel the lower back press into the towel, and thus the space disappears.

- Perform exercise on a chair, with hamstrings parallel to the floor, knees bent at 90 degrees, and feet grounded.

Tilting Hip Side to Side

- Supine, with spine in a neutral position—press one side of hip into the floor; allow the opposite side of hip to naturally lift. Move back and forth from sitting bone to sitting bone.

Sway Tail to Ribs

- Without moving the upper body, reach your tailbone toward one side of your ribs. Repeat on the other side.

Tailbone Curl and Release on All Fours

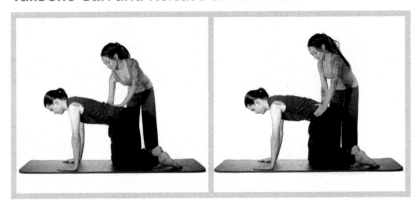

STARTING POSITION

On hands and knees, torso facing parallel to the floor, hands aligned with the shoulders, and knees aligned with the hips. Neutral spine from tailbone to top of the head, elbows soft, with inside of the elbows facing each other. *If assisting, stand beside client and place both hands on their hips. Guide the hips into an anterior tilt, with one hand placed on the lumbar and the other hand on the stomach to suggest maintaining the navel slightly pulled in.*

EXERCISE

- Inhale to lengthen tailbone.

- Push air out from the navel to curl tailbone around and down toward the floor. Energy goes where breath goes. Movement goes where energy and breath go.

- Repeat.

EMPHASIS

- Perform an *upside down* Pelvic Rock, focusing on *only* pelvic bowl rocking.

- Maintain length in spine and keep a slight chin nod.

IMAGERY

- Imagine stretching your tail to touch the wall, then drawing a line with your tail from the wall toward the space in between your knees.

- Visualize a bowl of water placed in the broad space in between your shoulder blades. Perform the exercise without moving the bowl at all.

AVOID

- overexaggerating the movement. Only move from tailbone.

- gripping trapezius and sinking rhomboids.

- hyperextending elbows with inside of elbows facing front.

- overloading wrists.

- dropping or extending head and neck away from neutral spine.

- fast, jerky movements.

REPETITION

- As needed, as preferred.

MODIFICATION

- For wrist pathologies, perform exercise on forearms.

- For shoulders or knee pathologies, use Pelvic Rock instead.

PROGRESSION

- Twist head side to side while performing the movement.

Groin to gut gateway

Visualize the pelvis as a bowl: When you carry that bowl, do you carry it in a level fashion, or are you "spilling your guts"? Simply practicing a walk with a level pelvic bowl can realign the body above and below. I often remember the Ida Rolf instruction to walk and stand with head up and waist back...remembering to keep that waist back accomplishes much the same thing as leveling the bowl.

I've been suggesting to students and clients lately that an "awakening" posture is to *try* (there, I said it, Rob!) to allow the genitals to move down and forward: Put your genitals out front but toward the ground...imagine they are on display! Next, find your belly button and pull it up and back at the same time as you pull your genitals down and forward. When you find this posture, I believe you're opening that gate between the groin and the gut, and allowing an energetic flow that may have been asleep for quite some time.

Just as we practiced standing and working to create balance between the feet, we can also work to find balance between the hips. Clearly, we need to begin with balanced feet, but allow yourself to examine in a mirror whether the hips seem balanced: Is one hip higher or further forward? Does one side of the back feel tighter? Simply working to note such an imbalance, then experimenting to correct that imbalance, can often change the way the hips work.

I also enjoy working with a lateral flexion. Maintaining the longest and straightest line I can find, I work to tighten one side of the body while lengthening the other side in lateral flex. As I'm fused from T10 to L3, this doesn't actually happen as much as I want.

On the other hand, when I'm faithful to this movement, my back feels much freer!

Image: Carry a level pelvic bowl through life.

Simple: Keep the groin downforward while the belly button stays upback.

Complex: Laterally flex (side to side), paying attention to the entire line, all the way to anchored inner arches, and to the movement of the head in lateral flexion.

Assisted Sacrum Release

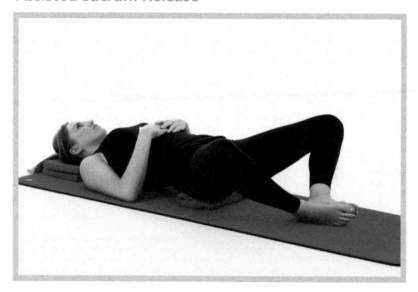

STARTING POSITION

Lie semi-supine with head resting on supportive pillow, allowing neck to remain long both front and back. Knees are bent and feet flat, hip width apart, with pressure balanced between heels and toes. Arms relaxed by your side and hands placed lightly along the bottom of ribcage. Lift and place sacrum onto a 5 inch (12 cm) inflatable ball so it is just above tailbone.

- Breathe in "slow and low," aiming to fill abdominal cavity between top of the pelvis and base of the ribcage.

- Trickle the air in to allow time to send it throughout the abdominal region and into base of the pelvis.

- As the air travels deep, think and feel for the weight of the sacrum on the ball while ribcage lifts into your hand.

- At the top of your inhalation, pause for a few seconds and think and feel for tension around pelvis.

- Begin a slow exhalation, targeting the areas that feel tight and restrictive to the breath, asking them to relax.

- Use the full exhalation to make sacrum feel heavier on the ball and thighs sinking into their sockets.

EMPHASIS

- Feel heaviness throughout sacrum and pelvis from back to front.

- Release the tension to increase the *flow of breath*.

- Relax into the posture and keep the body heavy to the floor, including shoulders.

IMAGERY

- Visualize sacrum as a filled water balloon. As you exhale, see the water balloon changing shape under the pressure of the firm ball.

AVOID

- allowing knees to collapse wide to begin with, keep them hip width apart, and focus on thighs being heavy.

REPETITION

- At least four "slow and low" breaths.

MODIFICATION

- If the position is too uncomfortable, consider using a rolled-up towel, to a thickness which is tolerable. Lift and place sacrum onto the rolled-up towel so it is just above tailbone.

PROGRESSION

- Consider lengthening the line further and reaching arms higher above head while allowing knees to release out wide.

Assisted Lower Abdominal Release

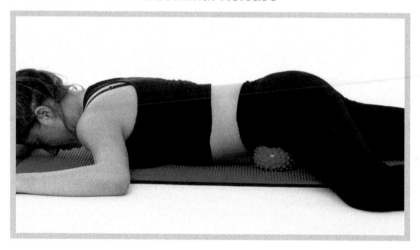

STARTING POSITION

Lie prone. Rest forehead on a pillow so neck can stay long, front and back. Keep nose clear of the floor.

EXERCISE

Abduct a leg out to the side, bringing knee up and resting the inside of the knee on the floor. Lift the same side pelvis slightly and place 5 inch (12 cm) inflatable ball underneath, just inside and below the iliac crest. Once the ball is in place, gently roll the pelvis around, up and over the ball, so that your intention is to move down, inside the ilium.

- Breathe in "slow and low," aiming to fill abdominal cavity between top of the pelvis and base of the ribcage.

- Trickle the air in to allow time to send it throughout the abdominal region and into the location of the ball.

- As the air travels deep, think and feel for the weight of the pelvis on the ball.

- At the top of your inhalation, pause for a few seconds and think and feel for any restrictions in the pelvic area.

- Begin a slow exhalation, targeting the areas that felt tight and restrictive to the breath, letting the restriction release.

- Use the full exhalation to make the restrictions smooth and pelvis even heavier on the ball.

EMPHASIS

- Feel heaviness throughout pelvis and more openness at the front.

- Release the tension to increase the *flow of breath*.

- Try to relax into the posture and use your breath to release the discomfort in pelvis.

IMAGERY

- Visualize the hipbone as a spoon. Gently scrape peanut butter off the inside of the spoon.

- As you exhale, see the ball gently sink into the pelvis, rolling into the peanut butter and smoothing it out!

AVOID

- allowing pelvis and lower back to lift too high.

- using a ball hard enough to create pain when you try to allow your weight to release over it.

REPETITION

- At least four "slow and low" breaths.

MODIFICATION

- If the position is too uncomfortable, consider using a rolled-up towel, to a thickness which is tolerable. Roll the towel up into a spherical shape as best as possible and apply pressure gently on to it as described for the ball above.

PROGRESSION

- Consider lengthening the line further and reaching arms higher above head and/or straightening knee out to the side.

Butterfly

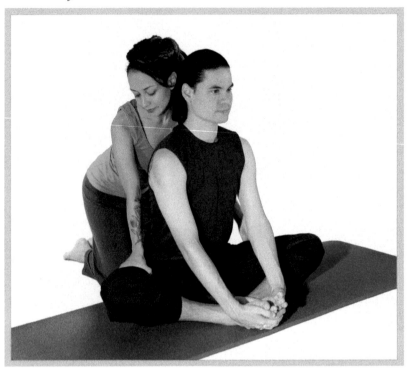

STARTING POSITION

Sitting upright on the floor. Soles of feet together and knees apart.

EXERCISE

- Inhale to pelvic floor. Expand pelvic floor and adductors, as if stretching the muscles from the inside of the body.

- Exhale, releasing the breath to make space. Hinge forward at hip and lower the body between legs toward the floor.

- Front and back of the body is lengthened, with shoulders relaxed.

- Adductors lengthen; knees reach down and out to the side as spine lowers.

EMPHASIS

- Pause at a point of stretch; breathe down into pelvic floor.
- Release and rise to return to starting position. Repeat.

IMAGERY

- Visualize your legs as butterfly wings.
- Spine elongates toward the sun.

AVOID

- pushing or forcing legs down.
- rounding shoulders forward.

REPITITION

- At least four 'low and slow' breaths.

MODIFICATION

- To elongate spine, place a blanket or pillow under sitting bones.
- To reduce adductor stretch, prop blankets and/or pillows underneath both knees.

PROGRESSION
Single Leg Butterfly

- One knee bent and out to the side; sole of foot presses against adductor of opposite leg.
- Opposite knee extends to the front.
- Lower upright spine toward the floor, as low as comfortably possible.

Supine Butterfly

- Perform stretch with torso lying face up on the floor. Prop under the knees if necessary.

- For too much discomfort in the spine, prop a pillow or blanket under the torso, keeping tailbone on the floor.

- Arms rest out to the sides of body.

Prone Single Leg Raise

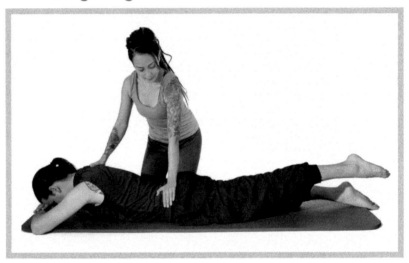

STARTING POSITION

Lie face down on the floor, legs extended and hip width apart, and hands under forehead. *When assisting, kneel beside the client, one hand stabilizing the shoulder, the other hand lightly pressing the posterior superior iliac spine (PSIS) to the floor as the client extends and floats the leg on the same side.*

EXERCISE

- Inhale to expand ribs, laterally and front to back.

- Exhale to press one ASIS down into ground.

- Inhale; leg rises off the ground while knee stays extended.

- Exhale and float leg back down.

EMPHASIS

- Focus on initiating the stretch from the front plane of the body.

- Stabilize pelvic bowl, emphasizing the lengthening from psoas and iliacus.

- Shoulders and upper torso remain relaxed.

IMAGERY

- Visualize your leg growing longer from your hip bone, stretching to reach your foot to the wall behind you.

- Imagine arrows shooting from the front of your hip through your leg and foot to the wall.

AVOID

- tensing the upper torso.

- squeezing the glutes and hamstrings to make the movements.

- lifting the ASIS off the floor or lifting legs too high off the floor. It is not about height, it is about length. The legs will lift as an afterthought.

REPETITION

- As long as needed or wanted.

MODIFICATION

- Place a blanket under the belly or hips to support lumbars and lengthen spine.

- For hyperextended knee, shorten the lever by bending knee at 90 degrees.

- For tensed upper extremities, reverse the breath—inhaling to begin, and exhaling to execute the movement.

PROGRESSION

- Allow leg to float out to side with the lift.

Gut center

Several years ago one of my students who is also a yoga teacher suggested that, frankly, we could all stay in healthy bodies if we'd only twist, laterally flex, and forward/backward flex and extend frequently. I follow this advice, and can tell it works for me. I'm reminded that, for me, what I call a "Willow X" exercise allows me to incorporate any of these four motions: twisting, then moving the trunk side to side, then bending both forward and backward. As I allow my arms to stay at least shoulder level and hopefully higher, I create an "X" with my body; then I move it, wherever I can explore. These four simple movements keep me flexible. I use small weights, and experiment with moving through other planes besides those four specific directions...that's why I think of it as a willow. Sometimes I use a stretching strap, put it behind my back, and find new directions for that willow to bend as well.

The yoga posture known as "pigeon" is one of my favorite psoas stretches. Kneel on the floor; then lengthen one leg behind you while sitting on the heel of the other foot. While keeping that back leg long, imagine you can stretch your upper body up, back, and into an arched extension while keeping the long leg's hip grounded into the floor. Now, allow yourself to explore: By turning your head and trunk away from the anchored longer leg, you're getting a good stretch for that psoas muscle. Breath is, of course, still important!

I'm also enjoying what I think of as a forward bend where I stand about 16 inches (40 cm) from a wall, facing the wall. I then place my head on the wall, and slowly slide the back of it down the wall toward the floor. When I reach my limit (and everyone's limit is in a different spot), I next focus on pushing my low back toward the ceiling *while* I'm sliding my head down the wall. For extra credit, turn the toes in and keep your weight in the inner arches. Delicious! When I'm traveling and don't have time for many stretches, I like to spend about one minute in this position, breathing and stretching.

Most simply, I'm advising self and others frequently to go through life and activities of daily living by imagining we can keep our waist back, more and more of the time. I find this simple cue invites me to activate my psoas in a relaxed fashion with every step.

CUES

Image: Keep the waist back in activities of daily living.

Simple: Pigeon pose from yoga.

Complex: Flex and extend forward and back in a segment-by-segment forward and back undulation of the entire spine. Move slowly and breathe!

Assisted Abdominal Release

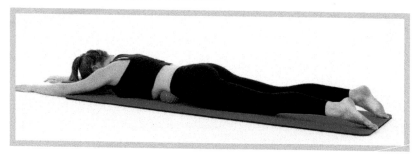

STARTING POSITION

Lie prone, and start by supporting your weight through your forearms. Lift and lower abdominal cavity onto a 5 inch (12 cm) inflatable ball so that the ball starts at the solar plexus. Ease your weight onto it, slowly making sure not to steal your breath.

- Breathe in "slow and low," aiming to fill abdominal cavity between the top of pelvis and the base of ribcage.

- Trickle the air in to allow time to send it throughout the abdominal region and into the location of the ball.

- As the air travels deep, think and feel for the weight of the stomach on the ball.

- At the top of your inhalation, pause for a few seconds and think and feel for any restrictions throughout.

- Begin a slow exhalation, targeting the ball and asking the body to melt over it further.

- Stay in this location for four breaths; then roll over the ball so that it travels down the lateral line of the rectus abdominis, starting on the left-hand side.

- Stop off anywhere you identify a restriction, and breathe into it.

- Repeat in each restriction for four breaths.

- Roll the ball as low as the inguinal line before going across to the right side and traveling back up.

EMPHASIS

- Feel heaviness throughout the abdominal cavity.

- Release the tension to increase the *flow of breath.*

- Try to relax into the posture and use your breath to release the discomfort in the abdomen.

- Make sure to travel around the abdominal region in a clockwise direction (down on your left and up on your right).

- Visualize picking up a large inflated gym ball, holding it between both hands. Imagine what would happen to that ball if you were to press it down onto a firm medicine ball. See how it distorts in shape and melts over the medicine ball. Aim to achieve the same, relaxed feeling in the abdominals as you lie over the ball at various points.

AVOID

- using a hard ball so you can allow your weight to release over it without creating pain.

REPETITION

- At least four "slow and low" breaths at each stricture.

MODIFICATION

- If the position is too uncomfortable, consider using a rolled-up towel, to a thickness which is tolerable.

PROGRESSION

- Consider lengthening the line further and reaching the arms higher above the head and/or straightening knee and leg out behind.

Self Abdominal Release

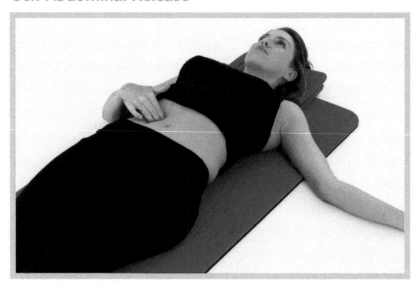

STARTING POSITION

Lie supine with legs lengthened out long from hips and relaxed, hip width apart. Place arms relaxed, and open out to the side with palms facing the ceiling to allow shoulders to widen. Head rests on supportive pillow, allowing neck to remain long both front and back.

EXERCISE

- Start by sinking your fingertips in, just below the inferior border of your last rib, on your left hand side, near to the lateral border of rectus abdominis, and ease the fingertips down with the intention of reaching the spine center from the front. Feel for any restrictions.

- Breathe in "slow and low," aiming to reach your fingertips.

- As the air travels deep, think and feel for the fingertips being gently lifted.

- At the top of your inhalation, pause for a few seconds and try to think and feel for any restrictions throughout.

- Begin a slow exhalation, targeting your touch and asking the tissue to let go.

- Stay in this location for four breaths, then continue down the lateral line of the rectus abdominis; stop off anywhere you identify a restriction.

- Repeat in each restriction for four breaths.

- Move down as far as the inguinal line before trying the opposite side.

EMPHASIS

- Release the tension to increase the *flow of breath*.

- Relax into the touch and use your breath to release the discomfort in the abdomen.

- Make sure to travel around the abdomen region in a clockwise direction (down on your left and up on your right).

IMAGERY

- Visualize the abdominals like a large gymnastic crash mat, ready to absorb the load of someone landing on it. As you apply pressure with your fingertips, aim to keep the abdominals relaxed so that the pressure is absorbed appropriately, as that mat would do.

AVOID

- pressing too hard, too quickly—coax the tissue release with slow and gentle pressure through the layers.

REPETITION

- At least four "slow and low" breaths at each stricture.

- If using your fingertips is too uncomfortable, consider using a ball and applying pressure with your palm over it.

PROGRESSION

- Consider lengthening the line further using your opposite hand for release and reaching the same side arm higher above the head as well as straightening the knee out behind.

Baby Cobra

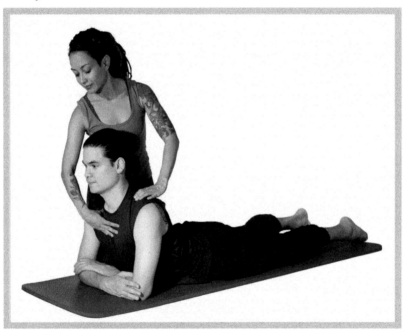

STARTING POSITION

Lie prone, with legs extended and forehead on the floor. Elbows and forearms are on the floor, beside the body. *If assisting, kneel besides the client. One hand guides the shoulders to round back, as the fingers and palm of the other hand on the sternum spreads the shoulders away from the front to suggest an open chest.*

EXERCISE

- Inhale; press forearms against the floor to lift the upper torso.
- Open chest, with scapulae relaxed back and down.
- Exhale; chin nod slightly.
- Rest in the pose.
- Inhale; reach from solar plexus a little more.
- Exhale; return to rest in the pose.

EMPHASIS

- Initiate the breath from solar plexus.
- Lightly pull navel in and nod chin to elongate spine.

IMAGERY

- Inhale; draw a line from your solar plexus on the floor up and toward the wall in front of you.
- Slide shoulder blades into your hip pockets.
- Imagine you are a proud Sphinx sitting comfortably on the sands.

AVOID

- sinking the body in between the scapulae.
- hyperextending neck back, thus jamming head into shoulders.
- allowing pelvic bowl and stomach to hang on the floor.

REPETITION

- Five deep breaths into solar plexus.

MODIFICATION
Turtle

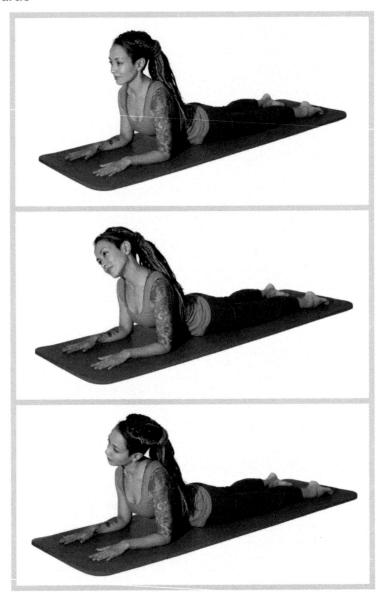

- Starting position at Baby Cobra pose...

- Visualize yourself as a turtle, with head out of shell, to slowly open and look around at the world.

- Turn only head to gaze behind. Repeat opposite side.

- Tilt ear to shoulder, then roll down, traveling chin to chest, toward opposite side. Repeat.

PROGRESSION
Somersaulting Turtle

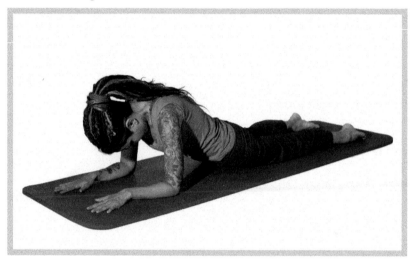

- Starting position as above.

- Inhale to expand lungs as you lift head out of your shell to look around at the world.

- Exhale to deflate and soften chest; then draw a line with your nose toward navel, curling your head under chest.

- Pushing your forearms to the floor, to curve the spine in between your shoulder blades.

- Inhale; resume starting position. Repeat.

Gut to heart gateway

The more we get clients, and self, to pay attention to breath, the healthier they can become. Remember, simply learning to breathe in and out at a rate of about six times per minute enhances heart rate variability and lessens many problems in the body, including arthritis and inflammation, diabetes, and heart conditions. To practice modified breathing I suggest to clients that they can count how many beats it takes them to inhale; then simply try to make a longer and slower inhale with succeeding breaths. If they work a bit, they might start at an in-breath of five or six, and work up to ten or twelve. The next difficulty: for many of us, that long, slow in-breath invites a rush of air out; the out-breath must happen quickly. No problem! Simply take that long, slow in-breath; then a rush of out-breath and a quick in-breath before a nice, slow out-breath. Repeating a sequence of slow in, fast out and in, slow out, fast in and out, back to slow in...etc. This sequence trains us to take in and allow more nourishment.

Further: If we can learn to breathe in to a satisfying count, but breathe out for a slightly longer count, doesn't it make sense that we're cleaning the lungs and exchanging oxygen more fully? I suggest that one monitors their in-breath; then try to make the out-breath go four counts longer. If we take a mild pause as well at the end of the breath, we're creating further health. I believe this breathing rate gives one a truly deep, cleansing oxygen exchange instead of the shallow lack of oxygenation too many of us are guilty of using instead. If we return to the healthy breathing rate which will enhance HRV, could we breathe in for a count of four and out for a count of five or six, with slight pauses at the top and bottom of the breath?

The intercostal muscles and serratus muscles are tremendously important; both stabilize ribs and inhibit the expansion of the ribcage. Stretching arms out of the ribcage begins to open the ribs and allow more breath to move through the chest. I continue to explore that "Willow X"; simply spreading my legs as I stand, raising arms, then allowing the body to twist, turn, and move all six star points around in space.

Look at that diaphragm muscle as the ceiling of the stomach and the floor of the heart. What sort of foundational floor does your heart have? Are the hiatuses or holes in the floor/ceiling too loose or tight? Does energy flow through? Do the heart and gut talk to each other through their hiatuses, or do they argue and refuse to communicate?

Pay attention in your own world to that which "takes your breath away"—perhaps a person, a situation, a place, or an attitude you find yourself holding. Simply realizing we're holding our breath, then choosing to do something about it, is a great start to changing the entire body.

CUES

Image: Simple attention to breath.

Simple: "Willow X" movement work, in every direction.

Complex: Self breath awareness—what "takes your breath away"?

Assisted Solar Plexus Opening Release

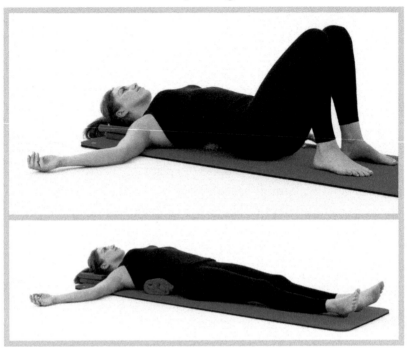

STARTING POSITION

Lie semi-supine with knees bent and feet flat, hip width apart, with pressure balanced between the heels and toes. Hold arms relaxed and open out to the side with palms facing the ceiling to allow the shoulders to widen. The head rests on a supportive pillow, allowing the neck to remain long both front and back. Lift and lower the thorax onto a 5 inch (12 cm) inflatable ball so that the ball is underneath and in line with the bottom of your breastbone/solar plexus. The correct position makes the solar plexus feel high up to the sky and bottom of the ribcage flared open.

EXERCISE

- Take a moment to explore and relax over the ball. Comfort in this posture can take a while to achieve and is largely dependent on how inflated the ball is—start off with it quite flat!

- Allow legs and pelvis to feel heavy into the floor and arms to relax out wide, allowing scapulae to connect with the floor.

- Breathe in "slow and low," aiming to reach your abdomen. Trickle the air in to allow time to send it throughout the abdominal region.

- As the air travels deep, think and feel for the weight of the trunk on the ball.

- At the top of your inhalation, pause for a few seconds and think and feel for any restrictions throughout.

- Begin a slow exhalation, targeting those restrictions and asking the body to melt further over the ball.

- Stay in this location for four breaths.

EMPHASIS

- Release the tension to increase the *flow of breath*.

- Relax into the ball and use your breath to release the discomfort in the thorax.

IMAGERY

- Visualize the spine laid on the floor like a bike chain, where each vertebra is a link in the chain. Now see the ball as the large cog; placing it under the spine lifts the chain off the floor, as the vertebrae roll up and over the ball.

AVOID

- staying on the ball if it's too uncomfortable and taking your breath away—come off and start with a towel!

REPETITION

- At least four "slow and low" breaths.

- If using the ball is too uncomfortable, revert to a rolled-up towel.

- Alternate tool: Place two tennis balls in a sock and place them on each side of the spinal bones.

PROGRESSION

- Consider lengthening the line further by taking both your arms and legs long away from the thorax.

Mermaid

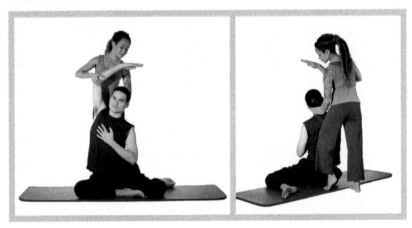

STARTING POSITION

Seated upright on the floor, prop sitting bones on pillow or blanket if necessary. Shoulders resting on top of the ribcage, fingertips lightly touching the floor, and legs in Z-position or cross-legged. *If assisting, stand behind client with their spine in side flexion, one hand holding the forearm of their extended arm. The other hand supports the head while the knee gently presses the client's back to maintain an open frontal plane.*

EXERCISE

- Place left palm on right side of ribcage.

- Inhale; expand the front, side, and back of the base of ribcage, fully challenging the diaphragm.

- Turn right arm out and raise toward the ear, fingers to the ceiling.

- Press right hip down while reaching the right line of the body beyond fingertips.

- Keep this arm parallel to ear, exhale, and flex spine toward left side of the body.

- Inhale into right side of the ribcage.

- Exhale; spine returns upright, with lower right arm down to the floor.

- Release left hand. Repeat on other side.

EMPHASIS

- Initiate the movements from diaphragm.

- Create and maintain space between ribs and hips throughout the exercise. Feel ribcage expand under the palm.

- Shoulders remain rested down and away from ears.

IMAGERY

- Create one long reach from the ground to sitting bone, through side of the body, into fingertips and toward the sky.

- Inhale; imagine inflating the balloon under your ribs. Feel the balloon expand and push your palm.

- Fan your ribs to open and close with every breath.

- Draw a rainbow from the ceiling toward the other side of the body.

- Form a bow-shape with spine. Explore the entire length of the bow.

AVOID

- allowing shoulders to rise up to ears.

- slouching or resting all the weight of the torso into opposite side.

- shortening waist and allowing opposite hip hikes off the floor.

- dropping head to opposite shoulder.

REPETITION

- Four repetitions, each side.

MODIFICATION

- Perform the exercise sitting straight on a chair, legs parallel to the floor, knees at 90 degrees, and feet grounded on the floor. As one arm floats up, the other hand holds the side edge of the chair.

PROGRESSION

- Allow the head to join in the movement, drawing circles into and away from the upper arm.

Heart Circles

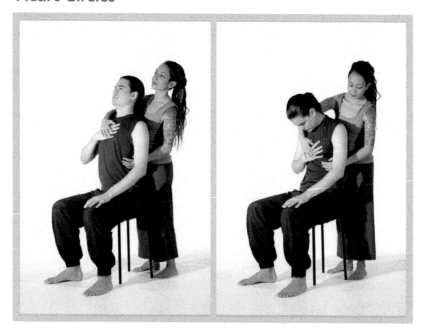

STARTING POSITION

Seated upright on a chair, legs parallel to the floor, knees at 90 degrees and feet grounded on the floor, shoulders resting on top of the ribcage, and hands resting on thighs. *If assisting, stand behind the client, one hand on the sternum, the other on the side of the ribcage to drive the upper torso into a circle drawing pattern.*

EXERCISE

- Place one hand on sternum.

- Inhale; expand the front of diaphragm, pressing sternum to palm.

- Shift and circle sternum to one side of torso.

- Exhale; round chest back and continue circling to other side.

- Inhale; continue circular motion toward the front of diaphragm. Repeat.

EMPHASIS

- Initiate the movements from diaphragm.

- Keep lower torso stabilized.

- Feel ribcage expand under palm.

- Shoulders remain rested down and away from ears.

IMAGERY

- Lead with your heart, drawing circles around your body.

- Visualize a light shining from your heart center, creating a halo that surrounds the front, sides, and back of your heart center.

AVOID

- squeezing scapulae together and hyperextending spine.

- rounding shoulder forward and slouching spine.

- pushing too much or too hard in any movement.

REPETITION

- Five circles in both directions.

MODIFICATION

- Break down the movement. Inhale; nudge sternum forward. Exhale; curl sternum and round spine back.

- Continue with shifting sternum from side to side.

PROGRESSION

- Combine sternum moving forward, side, back, side.

Heart center

One of my favorite ways to reverse this fetal posture we all seem to have a bit of (whether from emotional difficulties, computer/driving/texting/detail work, or poor posture in general) is to simply use a bolster under my "heart hinge" as I lie on the floor, prop my spine open, and breathe. I've purchased a bench which allows me to anchor the feet as I open my heart. I can lay flat on this bench, allow just my head to fall back off the bench, and breathe. Next I move a bit further up the bench so neck and shoulders are off the bench and arching me backward, extending the trunk toward the floor, with breath. I work on down the spine, next opening the thoracic spinal bones above my heart, around my heart, below the heart, and on into the low back...each segment being invited to have yet another deep breath while extending my head, my spine, and even my arms. For me, this simple stretch invites opening of all the upper points of the star, from that diaphragmatic/psoas heart center. Due to my fusion, anywhere from T7 to L4 could use a good dose of opening; nearly *all* of us could benefit from this heart opening, however.

Perhaps you don't have or can't afford money or space for a bench like mine. Do you have a couch in your home? I'm also comfortable using the couch: I put my head on the arm of the couch, breathe, and stretch. Next I move a bit further off the couch so my neck is on the couch arm, and again breathe and stretch. Little by little, I move my body further and further down that couch arm and off the couch, making each spinal segment the fulcrum for that stretch. Eventually, I nearly somersault off the couch as I reach my low back... while it's good to open any hinges up and down the spine, the heart is often the most needed.

One of my simplest cues can be most complex... When I ask clients to go home and "lead with their heart," many interesting emotional reactions can occur. Simple, but profound.

CUES

Image: Lead with the heart through "activities of daily living" (ADLs).

Simple: Use a bolster or bench to "pop open" the heart hinge (and any others), with breath.

Complex: Head up, waist back, groin downforward, heart out, and stay mildly in the toes as often as you can remember and find.

Assisted Breastbone and Intercostals Release

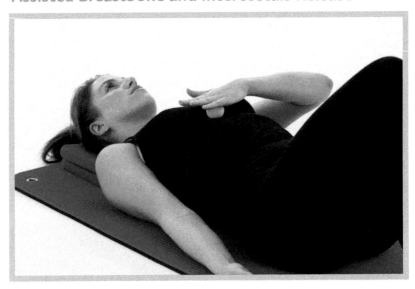

STARTING POSITION

Lie semi-supine with knees bent and feet flat, hip width apart. Keep pressure balanced between the heels and toes. Arms remain relaxed and open out to the side with palms facing the ceiling to allow shoulders to widen. Head rests on a supportive pillow, allowing neck to remain long both front and back. Place a small hard ball (racquet or squash ball) on breastbone, just below manubrium, and keep it in place with light pressure from the palm of one hand.

EXERCISE

- Apply gentle pressure through the ball and roll it in small circles in a clockwise direction. Pause at any points on the breastbone that feel sore and uncomfortable.

- Keeping the pressure on these points, breathe into abdomen.

- At the top of your inhalation, pause for a few seconds and think and feel for the restrictions and soreness.

- Begin a slow exhalation, targeting those restrictions and asking the body to let them release.

- Stay in this location for four breaths.

- Then move on to another point on the breastbone that "talks back" to you—another restriction.

- BE WARNED—THIS CAN BE SORE THE FIRST TIME IT IS DONE!

EMPHASIS

- Release the tension to increase the *flow of breath*.

- Allow the breastbone to open up fully, freeing the diaphragm underneath.

IMAGERY

- Visualize the breastbone as the peak of a badly pitched tent, collapsed to the floor.

- See the rolling of the breastbone as a way to break down any substance that is preventing the tent from lifting up high again.

- As you roll it out, you should feel it wanting to float up high.

AVOID

- applying so much pressure that it makes you hold your breath.

REPETITION

- Pause at each stricture for approximately four breaths.

MODIFICATION

- If you don't have a ball, or using one is too uncomfortable, make a light fist with one hand and apply gentle pressure with your knuckles.

PROGRESSION

- Consider lengthening the line further by taking an arm out and away from breastbone, *while* you keep your low back anchored into the floor.

Welcoming Arms, Hug Yourself

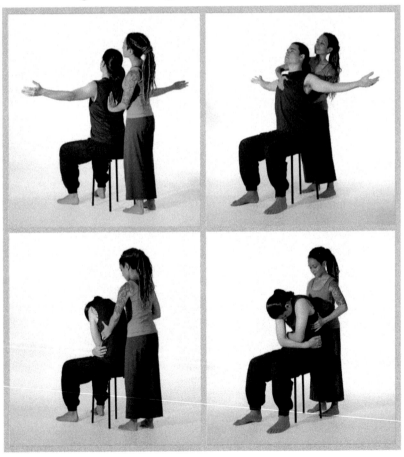

STARTING POSITION

Seated on the floor or chair, prop sitting bones on pillow or blanket if necessary. If on a chair, legs are hip width apart, knees relaxed at a 90 degree angle, and feet placed comfortably on the floor. Spine is elongated, shoulders relaxed, and arms down the side of the body; arms supinated, palms face forward. *If assisting: Stand behind the client.* **Welcoming arms:** *one hand on chest, other hand in between scapulae to guide sternum to move forward and up.* **Hug yourself:** *both hands by the sides of ribcage to pull upper torso back and down.*

EXERCISE

- Inhale to extend and expand the entire front of the body, giving freedom to lift and open chest; allow the breath to fill extended arms, hands, and fingertips as it reaches toward back of the body.

- Exhale; release the breath fully to curl thorax down, opening back.

- Float arms forward, wrap arms around front of the body, with elbows stacked on top of each other. Repeat.

EMPHASIS

- Initiate the movements from diaphragm, with breath.

- Maintain shoulders down and away from ears; arms float forward and back at chest level, yet below shoulder height.

- Allow thorax, spine, and head to follow the movement organically.

- Enjoy the movement!

IMAGERY

- Welcome yourself with arms open wide, then give yourself the biggest, warmest hug.

- Visualize your arms as wings spread as wide as possible, soaring above the clouds.

- Wrap the wings around your body, blanketing yourself from harm.

AVOID

- hyperextending arms.

- allowing shoulders to rise up to ears.

- slouching and hyperextending spine throughout the movement.

- taking yourself too seriously!

REPETITION

- Five hugs.

MODIFICATION

- Perform the exercise with elbows bent at 90 degrees and arms externally rotated so palms face forward.

- Inhale into chest and elbows to open and pull elbows/hands back gently; exhale, release, and bring elbows together.

PROGRESSION

- While hugging yourself, allow your body to twist side to side as you keep the lower back rounded back.

Heart to head gateway

For me, simply opening and paying attention to the restriction between the head and heart, that throat chakra area, is critical. We all know people who seem to live in their heads; totally intellectual, wanting the reasoning, the protocol, the "why" of whatever is being discussed. If we ask them to descend to their heart and check on feelings, we're often met with blank stares. How do we get someone who lives in their head to descend into their body and explore? Though we've started at the ground and worked our way up to the heavens, it's totally true that too many of us only reside in the head. Can we bring such folks into the full body? With attention and intention, yes.

This is a horrible and sometimes unfair generalization, but can you see some truth? I posit that survivors of sexual abuse often live in their heads more than in the rest of their body. Can you see the common sense of that theory? Can you see how something bad happening in the lower body would drive one higher? And can you also see how oral abuse could result in further restriction of the throat and a further tightening to the head?

Three techniques I rely on to help keep my throat chakra open: First, I hum a lot! Through the day, I hear a piece of music and a bit sticks with me; I repeat it over and over as I go about my work. I feel this simple humming, like a meditator's mantra or "Om," is causing energy to move through the throat.

Second, I love hanging by my fingers from doorway trims or any appropriately high support that allows me to open shoulder girdles while keeping my head upback, and breathing. I believe it's critical to get our shoulders and arms out of our necks and throats in order to allow this energy flow to rise toward the head. Perhaps one is too short to reach the top of the doorway trim; perhaps a short stool or some such tool will allow the correct space. If not, a good alternative is to simply lift one's body, using the arms by placing hands on a table or counter, then letting the spine hang down long by use of those arms while pushing the body up. I see it as hanging the spine from the shoulders and neck instead of hanging the shoulders off the spine and neck.

And, last, I've realized that finding a proximal hinge and asking for movement from it often changes the strength of a stretch. I get better bodywork results often by asking for a knee or elbow movement instead of a foot or hand movement, moving from the proximal joint instead of the distal one. Therefore, I enjoy standing, putting my elbows above my head while hands stay on the back of the head, and tugging elbows upback toward the ceiling in a way that I feel them pull out of my shoulders, then out of my mid back, low back, and finally out of my legs and feet! With breath, of course.

CUES

Image: Hum, or make Om sounds…move energy through the throat!

Simple: Hang the shoulders from the spine *and* the spine from the shoulders—whether hanging from something or putting hands on a counter and pushing self up.

Complex: Arm stretches from the elbow; use proximal joints for stretches instead of distal ones.

Assisted Pectoralis and Subclavian Release

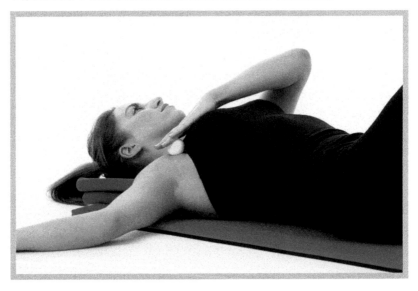

STARTING POSITION

Lie semi-supine with knees bent and feet flat, hip width apart, with pressure balanced between heels and toes. Arms are relaxed and open out to the side with palms facing the ceiling to allow shoulders to widen. Head rests on a supportive pillow, allowing neck to remain long both front and back. With the palm of the opposite hand, place a small, hard ball on the sternoclavicular joint of one side; then gently roll it down so it sits just underneath the inferior border of the clavicle.

EXERCISE

- Apply gentle pressure through the ball and roll it slowly along length of clavicle, then down onto pectoralis.

- Pause at any points along clavicle and across pectoralis that feel sore and uncomfortable.

- Keeping the pressure on at these points, breathe into abdomen.

- At the top of your inhalation, pause for a few seconds and think and feel for the restriction and soreness.

- Begin a slow exhalation, targeting those restrictions, and asking the body to let them release.

- Stay in this location for four breaths.

- Then move on to another point along this line that "talks back" to you—another restriction.

- BE WARNED—THIS CAN BE SORE THE FIRST TIME IT IS DONE!

- Release the tension to increase the *flow of breath.*

- Allow the top of the thorax to open and help release length up the neck.

IMAGERY

- Visualize the clavicle as a swing bridge that has been bolted too tight and can't swing. See the rolling on the clavicle and pectoralis as a way of loosening the bolts that are preventing the bridge from swinging. We want the clavicle to swing with the arm movement, freeing up the neck.

AVOID

- applying so much pressure that it makes you hold your breath.

REPETITION

- At each stricture for approximately four breaths.

MODIFICATION

- If you don't have a ball or using one is too uncomfortable, use the tips of your fingers.

PROGRESSION

- Consider lengthening the line further by taking an arm out away from the breastbone in a large circle, opening up the clavicle and rotating the head the opposite way.

Lion

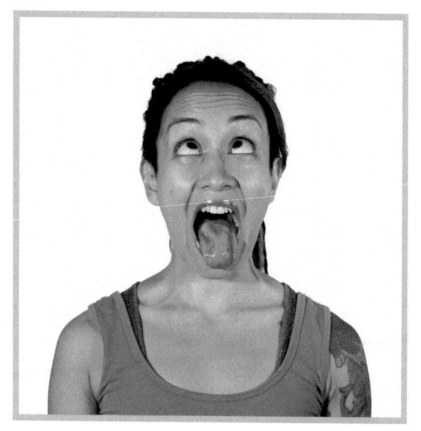

STARTING POSITION

Seated comfortably—cross-legged on the floor, prop sitting bones on pillow or blanket if necessary; may use a chair or kneel instead. Spine upright, body at ease, shoulders relaxed on top of the ribcage, and hands resting on lap. Face and jaw are relaxed.

EXERCISE

- Inhale at starting position; exhale, open mouth wide, and stick out tongue while eyes are looking in between eyebrows simultaneously.

- Let out a long, audible sigh.

- Inhale; return to starting position. Repeat.

EMPHASIS

- Open mouth as wide as possible and stick tongue out as far as possible.

- Exhale and sigh until the last drop of breath before inhaling again.

- Have fun with it!

IMAGERY

- Imagine you are a baby lion letting out your very first roar, as long and as loud as possible.

AVOID

- tensing the rest of the body.

- taking yourself too seriously.

- thinking that it is lame and/or silly (just try it!).

REPETITION

- Three times.

MODIFICATION
Yawn

- Inhale; open mouth as wide as possible.

- Exhale and sigh, then close mouth.

PROGRESSION

- Avoid the feeling of embarrassment that comes with it. Let it out proud! Explore the feelings.

Head center

Sometimes I'll do neck rolls where I invite myself to believe that any one of the many segments of the spine is the only segment that moves the neck. Imagine one can only roll their neck from the occiput/c1 junction...work slowly in both directions, trying to stabilize every other vertebral segment in the body. Then work down one or two segments: What happens when you try to roll the neck from the c3/4 junction? Remember to isolate that segment and try to move the rest of the spine as little as possible. What about t6? l1? Can you act, feel, and believe these are the only spinal segments that move the neck? Many of us have one or two neck joints we like "cracking," often to distraction. While creating that movement may not be a bad idea, creating hyper-movement in one segment/joint seems to suggest hypo-mobility directly above and below, and that's to be avoided. Creating length and flexibility in the neck, especially upper, adds energy and movement to the head but, if we do this well, we find more stretch along that long, deep line we've been chasing. So, we're lifting the head, but lifting it off the body.

Be aware that *any* neck rolling from *any* hinge will work *all* hinges! The idea in that particular bit was to get you thinking about twisting, flexing, and extending from the heart hinge...a worthy goal indeed! But why let that be the only focus? Explore *every* hinge.

Remember two concepts here: First, that as many of us work with computers, or drive, or text too often; we've created a forward neck and therefore a shortened front of neck and hypertonic back of neck. Also remember the concept that unresolved thought forms can collect at the back of the neck. Allow yourself to lift the head upback as you release the negativity that can collect in this area.

CUES

Image: Lift self upback from the bald spot/tonsure at top/back of head.

Simple: c1/2 neck rolls.

Complex: Involve the whole body in neck rolls. Believe any spinal segment can be the only segment that moves the head and all the rest must remain static.

Assisted Masseter Release

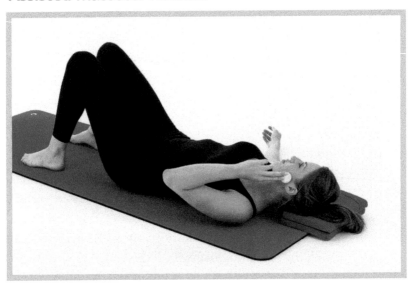

Lie semi-supine with knees bent and feet flat, hip width apart, with pressure balanced between heels and toes. Arms are relaxed and open out to the side with palms facing the ceiling to allow shoulders to widen. Head rests on a supportive pillow, allowing neck to remain long both front and back. With light pressure from the palm of your hand, place a small, hard ball on the masseter muscle.

EXERCISE

- Apply gentle pressure through the ball and roll it slowly in a clockwise motion. Pause at any points along the tissue that feel sore and uncomfortable.

- Keeping the pressure on at these points, breathe into abdomen.

- At the top of your inhalation, pause for a few seconds and think and feel for the restriction and soreness.

- Begin a slow exhalation, targeting those restrictions and asking the body to let them release.

- Stay in this location for four breaths.

- Then move on to another point along this line that "talks back" to you—another restriction.

- BE WARNED—THIS CAN BE SORE THE FIRST TIME IT IS DONE!

EMPHASIS

- Release the tension to increase the *flow of breath.*

- Allow the cranial bones to feel some release and opening.

IMAGERY

- Visualize the masseter muscle as a coiled spring. See the rolling of the muscle as a way of loosening the spring and making it sag. We want masseter tension to release so that the jaw feels relaxed.

AVOID

- applying so much pressure that it makes you hold your breath and clench your jaw!

REPETITION

- Pause at each restriction for approximately four breaths.

MODIFICATION

- If you don't have a ball or using one is too uncomfortable, use the tips of your fingers.

- Consider lengthening the line further by taking an arm out away from the breastbone and rotating the head long, the opposite way, to help open up the neck.

Crane and Dragon Neck

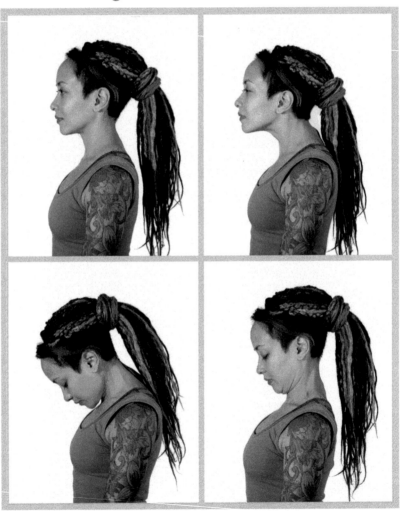

STARTING POSITION

Sitting, with spine long. Knees soft, legs hip width apart, and hands on hips.

EXERCISE

- While keeping head sitting directly on top of the shoulders, pull back of the head back.

- Breathe into the front of chest and neck, slightly lift chin up, and move head forward with a hooking movement, as if pulling yourself forward with your chin.

- Breathe out; expand the space in between each vertebrae as you pull the chin back into the back of neck by extending the top and back of head.

- Reverse the movement by curling head down, then circle upward, leading with nose.

- Pull the back of neck back to return to position.

EMPHASIS

- The rest of the body remains still and relaxed.

- The entire neck is fluid.

IMAGERY

- Imagine you are a bird scraping the ground for food.

- Visualize you are the bird scooping and drinking water.

AVOID

- allowing any tension in the body.

REPETITION

- Nine repetitions each way.

MODIFICATION
Rock the Kun Lun

- Rotate head from side to side; pause on each side and exhale.

- Drop shoulders while gazing as far behind you as possible.

- Continue by tilting head, ear to shoulder.

- Also pause as you tilt to one side and exhale, keeping face facing forward and eyes gazing downward to the ground.

- Three repetitions on each side, for both exercises.

- Can be done sitting on a chair.

PROGRESSION

- Draw an infinity symbol or horizontal figure 8 with the tip of your nose.

- Draw the symbol as small or as big as your neck permits, while the rest of the body is relaxed.

Head to heaven gateway

Ida Rolf often reinforced her one sure-fire cue to change bodies: "top of the head up, back of the waist back." It's easy to get the head on top, but too many of us do so by pulling the waist forward. Remember how an earlier cue was to suggest we go through life with the waist back? What happens when we ask the head to stay on top as well? It's difficult! Ask the waist to move back and the head will roll forward. Paying attention to both at once, and becoming the general instead of the foot soldier, allows us to experience energy into the head center. Energy equals circulation, nerve function, clear thinking, and joy.

Return to the idea of simply standing and exploring the concept that the neck can roll from many various levels in the spine: We can't keep a good head on our shoulders if we can't isolate up and down the line, and keep energy moving in all the hinges and restrictions. Any work that asks cervical spinal segments to create space and energy is time well spent.

These days I spend far more time on a computer than I used to do. I realize that it doesn't take me long to move into poor posture—head creeping forward, heart hinge shortening, and the entire body tensing and going fetal. I've realized that if I just stop, take a few minutes, extend my spine, and then grab the back of my head with both hands and pull the head down and forward *while* pushing the back of the neck and occiput up and back, while breathing, I can often reverse hours of poor posture and achievement mode. Simple to do, not easy to remember!

While this book isn't meant to endorse any particular mode or method, do consider the idea of craniosacral therapy, which posits that the bones of the cranium are meant to be moveable instead of fused. Clients with extreme headaches and tight craniums may want to consider cranial work to enhance what they can do for themselves.

I'm very happy encouraging my partner to use a rolled towel (a terry cloth robe belt works best for us) behind my head as I lie down. She simply tugs to create traction on my neck, and I'm able to cue her as to how much or how little traction to provide, while I'm breathing. Delicious!

CUES

Image: Become the general who watches from high above instead of the foot soldier who loses his head.

Simple: Remember the Ida Rolf admonition: top of the head up, back of the waist back.

Complex: Ask a partner to place a towel behind your neck/head while you lay on the floor. Give them instruction as to how much traction you enjoy, while you continue to breathe.

Last thought: Let go!

Assisted Suboccipital Muscles Release

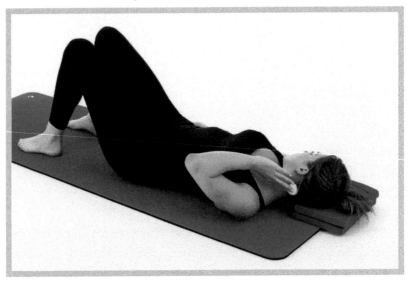

STARTING POSITION

Lie semi-supine with knees bent and feet flat, hip width apart, with pressure balanced between heels and toes. Arms are relaxed and open out to the side with palms facing the ceiling to allow shoulders to widen. Head rests on a supportive pillow, allowing neck to remain long both front and back. With light pressure from the palm of your hand or your fingertips, place a small, hard ball on base of occiput.

EXERCISE

- Apply gentle pressure through the ball and roll it slowly from lateral to medial.

- Pause at any points along the tissue that feel sore and uncomfortable.

- Keeping the pressure on at these points, breathe into abdomen.

- At the top of your inhalation, pause for a few seconds and think and feel for the restriction and soreness.

- Begin a slow exhalation, targeting those restrictions and asking the body to let them release.

- Stay in this location for four breaths.

- Then move on to another point along this line that "talks back" to you—another restriction.

- BE WARNED—THIS CAN BE SORE THE FIRST TIME IT IS DONE!

EMPHASIS

- Release the tension to increase the *flow of breath*.

- Allow the cranial bones some release and opening.

- Release the head from neck—giving it freedom again.

IMAGERY

- Visualize the skull resting on the neck like an olive on a cocktail stick. See the olive as sitting unevenly, with too much weight at the front and the stick piercing through the back. We want the olive balanced on the stick—as we want the head supported by the neck.

AVOID

- applying so much pressure that it makes you hold your breath and move away from the pain.

REPETITION

- Pause at each stricture for approximately four breaths.

MODIFICATION

- If you don't have a ball, or using one is too uncomfortable, use the tips of your fingers.

- Two soft smaller balls wrapped together in a stocking make another good tool.

- Consider lengthening the line further by turning the occiput away in the opposite direction.

Self Suboccipital Muscles Release

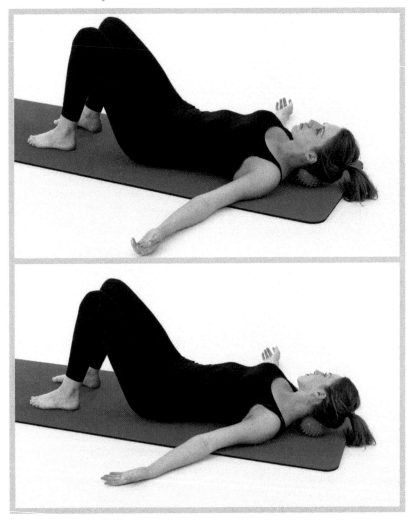

Lie semi-supine with knees bent and feet flat, hip width apart, with pressure balanced between heels and toes. Arms relax and open out to the side with palms facing the ceiling to allow shoulders to widen. Head rests on a 5 inch (12 cm) inflatable ball so that it sinks up and into the occiput area.

EXERCISE

- Apply gentle pressure through the ball and roll it slowly from side to side and up and down (chin nod to head back).

- Pause at any points along the tissue that feel sore and uncomfortable.

- Keeping the pressure on at these points, breathe into abdomen.

- At the top of your inhalation, pause for a few seconds and think and feel for the restriction and soreness.

- Begin a slow exhalation, targeting those restrictions and asking the body to let them release.

- Stay in this location for four breaths.

- Then move on to another point along this line that "talks back" to you—another restriction.

- BE WARNED—THIS CAN BE SORE THE FIRST TIME IT IS DONE!

EMPHASIS

- Release the tension to increase the *flow of breath*.

- Allow the cranial bones some release and opening.

- Release the head from the neck—giving it freedom again.

IMAGERY

- Visualize the skull like a gyroscope that's slowing down. Consider the head having a similar freedom of movement at the top of the spine.

AVOID

- applying so much pressure that it makes you hold your breath and move away from the pain.

REPETITION

- Pause at each restriction for approximately four breaths.

MODIFICATION

- If you don't have a ball, or using one is too uncomfortable, try rolling a tennis ball up in a towel and placing it loosely in the same place.

PROGRESSION

- Consider lengthening the line further by opening out both arms even further—reaching them wide of each other as you try your head movements: up, down, side to side.

Eye and Face Work

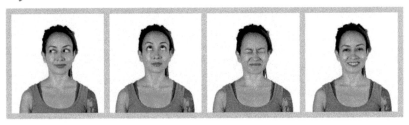

STARTING POSITION

Seated comfortably—cross-legged on the floor, prop sitting bones on pillow or blanket if necessary, or seated on a chair or kneeling if you prefer. Spine upright, body at ease, shoulders relaxed on top of the ribcage, and hands resting on lap; face and jaw are relaxed.

EYE EXERCISES

- Rotate eyes clockwise five times and counterclockwise five times.

- Gaze to the left and right. Repeat.

- Focus at the tip of the nose, then change focus to a point at the furthest distance possible.

FACE EXERCISES

- Tense the face muscles and clench the jaw, then open mouth wide into Lion. Repeat.

- Raise and then flex eyebrows. Repeat.

- Pucker lips and draw circles with your mouth.

- Make the angriest face, then release into the biggest smile!

EMPHASIS

- Have fun with it!

- Have a good laugh at/with yourself.

IMAGERY

- Dance with your eyes. Make shapes with them.

- Make the funniest, most expressive facial expressions.

AVOID

- taking yourself too seriously.

- thinking that it's lame and/or silly (just try it!).

REPETITION

- As many times as you like!

MODIFICATION

- Open mouth as wide as possible, exhale, and sigh, then close mouth.

PROGRESSION

- Allow your head to now explore as well as moving the facial muscles.

Appendix B

Stretches/Awareness that Incorporate More than One Center and Gateway

Remember my concept, shared often through the book, that one stretches a rubber band in more directions to create optimal stretches... In this appendix, Liz and I focus on moving centers and gateways further away from each other. While this appendix will be shorter, it's meant to encourage therapists to make it up! Create stretches that move the body longer and straighter, and that allow energy to flow through the entire being more fully... Open the head, heart, gut, and groin, but also create space in any and all areas that may be compressed, in longer lines of awareness.

With this concept in mind, revisit most of the cues and ideas we've shared in Appendix A. Can you see that, actually, most of what's been presented has already used the concept of bringing a stretching awareness to more than simply the one center or gateway that was featured in each segment? Especially if you visit Rob's "Progressions" in Appendix A, you'll see this lengthening and enhancing the length of lines of awareness. Any time we stretch and become aware of any center or gateway, we're already stretching up or down the lines further, whether we yet feel it or not. Whether suggested or not, as you review most exercises, much of the time one either sees a not-too-subtle invitation to join these stretches across and between various segments, or as you revisit and think about any of the stretch ideas, you can see how easy it would be to stretch that rubber band further. By moving *something else* up or down the line, you easily add more stretch to what's already been shown. This appendix will offer further guidance on ways to incorporate more of the centers and gateways into more of the stretches.

The same rules apply for these stretches as for all others. First, remember the breath can be the movement...don't feel you must achieve or overdo! As you stretch, remember that if breath can't reach an area, you're overdoing. Next, remember your stretch is meant to be an exploration, not an achievement. And add to these rules the idea that each stretch is designed to help you locate and join more and more of your centers and gateways into a longer and more open line.

Stretching ground to groin from groin and above

I've realized I get entirely different stretching work done if I lie on my back, then literally pull my big toe's lateral cuticle away from my sacrum. By simply adding the idea of also bringing the chin toward the chest so the back of the neck is long *while* keeping the low back downback, we're adding stretch and awareness all the way up and down the line—ground to groin, groin, and head, to name three participants.

Stretching ground to groin from head

Liz has alluded to this already, as have I. Simply walk mindfully, with awareness of toe and ankle hinges, and push off. This changes everything above, especially when we carry head up and waist back. And let me repeat how important I believe it is to find that Bubbling

Spring. I align my feet and try to match them; then I squat to comfort. Then I curl forward *slowly* with head reaching toward floor, and explore. If palms will reach the floor, that's great, but not necessary. Remember to keep the knees mildly flexed as you isolate and enjoy the stretch in your low and mid back.

Stretching gut from ground to groin and from head to heaven at the same time

Revisit my concept of a forward bend against a wall in Appendix A. Remember how we faced a wall, allowed the head to descend down that wall, then pushed the low back toward the ceiling? Remember how we then enhanced the stretch by turning the toes inward and pushing the inner arches into the floor? Can you see that this line encourages stretching of *everything*, but specifically that we're stretching gut, ground to groin, groin to gut, back of heart, and head to heavens?

Stretching head and heart from groin

Stand; clasp fingertips together pad to pad, then place one elbow behind the head and let the other land where it will. Now, bring that back elbow up to ceiling and pull both the elbow and head up and away from the low back and groin, or groin to gut. As you explore small circles with the elbow and head, the heart, gut to heart, gut, and groin to gut are all receiving a longer line stretch.

We could create such stretches for you all day; the point we wish to make with this appendix is that you can do the same! By simply thinking of any two or three, or more, points on this chart of nine centers and gateways, and then thinking how one could create space between such points, you will find, create, and use new stretches that haven't yet occurred to you. Good luck!

Introduction

This appendix is a compilation of exercises from four different movement modalities—yoga, dance, Pilates, and tai chi. Though different in terms and language, these practices share a significant amount of similarities. It's been fun to play with fusing ideas of different techniques into each exercise. Most importantly, this appendix brings Noah's bodymindcore into the exercises. Now this is when it gets interesting!

Take the biggest and best example to date: the pelvic floor. In yoga, we learn about the *bandha*, or lock. Bandhas are meant to be "locked" or contracted to block energy flow through the area, usually during inhalation or holding the breath. During exhalation, the retained energy is released and lightly rushed upward to the rest of the body. At the pelvic floor, we have the *mula bandha*, or root lock. It is meant to be locked to retain and then send a flow of energy upward to the rest of the body. Similarly, in tai chi and qi gong, there is Hui Yin, the acupuncture point located between the anus and the genitals, known to be gently contracted and pulled up to also lift energy upward through the body. In Pilates, we understand that pulling the pelvic floor up toward the navel will help strengthen what we commonly call core and stabilize our torso.

If, all across the board, schools and disciplines are saying the same things, then this action must be meant to be good for us, right? Well, here's the thing: We may be doing too much. Although the beliefs/facts/understanding behind it are good and have good intentions, we may have gone a little too far. We may be contracting so much that we no longer just retain and lift up energy—we block it completely... and we don't realize it. So when our knees start to hurt, we think they're weak. We do more squats and lunges to try strengthening them, but it doesn't work. Why not? Well, if we're tightening and contracting everywhere, how can energy flow to our knees and down to our feet?

It's becoming rare that we give our bodies the chance to let go. I don't mean to let go forever and always, but we shouldn't be teaching our students to tighten forever and always either. We need to look for the in-between and expand from there.

Take Noah's idea of imagining ourselves with a tail. If you were to look at other animals, it would be hard to find too many roaming the earth with their tails permanently sucked into their bodies. So what if we were to educate our students or clients to free their tails as well, without sticking our bottoms out nor dragging a heavy tail? What would it be like to have a tail that sways freely and stays relaxed? Have your students play with both actions—contract and release.

Teach your students to explore the many lines of the body. For example, even when they are tapping their toes, ask them about what's happening in their shoulders and neck. If they are too focused on staying in plank position, hands planted hard on the floor with strong arms, pelvic floor pulled up, and navel to spine, get them to notice their head jutted down toward the floor. Energy will no longer flow effectively and will only lead to pain and injury. Energy locked is energy blocked!

Train your students to stop focusing on just one or two areas in the body, because that is where *locking then blocking* happens. Instead, guide them to stretch from any and every area—to feel a line from the top of the head down to the tail. Then travel back up that line from the tip of the tail to the top of the head. Then run from fingertip to fingertip, sole to sole. Progress from tail to fingertips, top of the head to soles of the feet, tip of the tail to the front of the heart...the list can go on and on.

The idea of this appendix is not about taking and using only these exercises in the book in your classes or sessions. As Rob has said in Appendix A, these are just samples to spark curiosity of other modalities out there that may empower you and enhance your teachings. We intend to show how instead of contracting/pulling/locking bandhas and acupuncture points, Noah's idea of unlocking gateways between centers may be the key to creating a balanced body that is neither stiff nor loose, but resilient and pain free.

Bodymindcore within movement, incorporating multiple centers

Banana Stretch

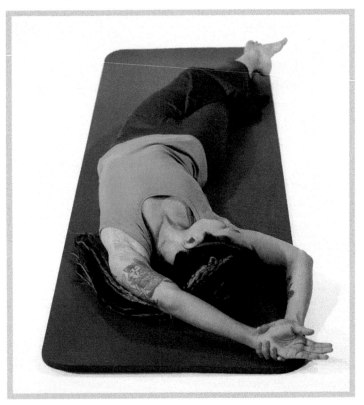

EXERCISE

Lie on the edge of the mat. Legs together, hands beside the body; cross leg one on top of the other, and bring the legs to the opposite corner of the mat.

- Float arms up to ears; hold wrist.

- Gently pull arm and reach to the same side of the mat.

- Inhale; reach both upper and lower extremities away from groin to gut.

- Exhale; release.

- Add flexion to the opposite side of the body as you inhale.

- Exhale; remain and rest in the position.

IMAGERY

- Creating the shape of a banana with your body!

AVOID

- sliding shoulders up to ears.

- anteriorly tilting hips and/or overarching lumbars.

GATEWAYS

Initiate the stretch from the gut center reaching down into groin to ground (reverse), *while* heart center opens and illuminates *with* the arms overhead to heart to head to heavens.

NOAH'S EXTRA

Keep the hips as close to the mat as possible, while keeping the cleanest lateral flexion you can manage. Where do *you* cheat?

Pelvic Clock

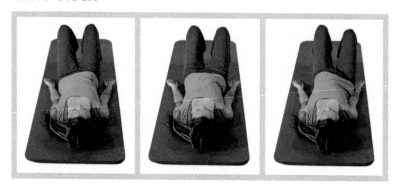

EXERCISE

Lie supine, soft, and lengthened on the floor. Knees bent and hip width apart (add soft ball or pillow to stabilize knees if necessary). Feet aligned with knees; heels 2–3 inches (5–8 cm) away from the sitting bones. Pelvis and spine are in a neutral position.

- Combine the Pelvic Rock, Tilting Hip Side to Side, and Sway Tail to Ribs (refer to Appendix A, pages 146–148).

- Inhale to anteriorly tilt, and continue to bring the pelvis toward PSIS on one side.

- Exhale to travel and trace the pelvis back down toward the sacrum, creating a posterior tilt or imprint of the spine; then back toward PSIS on the other side.

- Return to starting position; repeat and reverse the movement.

IMAGERY

- Draw a clock on your hips, pausing at 12 o'clock to 3 o'clock to 6 o'clock to 9 o'clock, then return to 12 o'clock.

- Move a bowl of water on top of your pelvic area around in a circle.

AVOID

- allowing knees to sway freely.

- stiffening chest and shoulders.

GATEWAYS

Ground to groin is stable while movement is initiated from the groin center and groin to gut. Heart center remains soft while heart to head reaches subtly toward head to heavens.

Remember my idea that we're all bound in our sexual centers? When we're serious about looking at our sexuality and its expression, this is a powerful piece of work. Can you allow sexual energy and feelings as you explore these cues?

Bridge

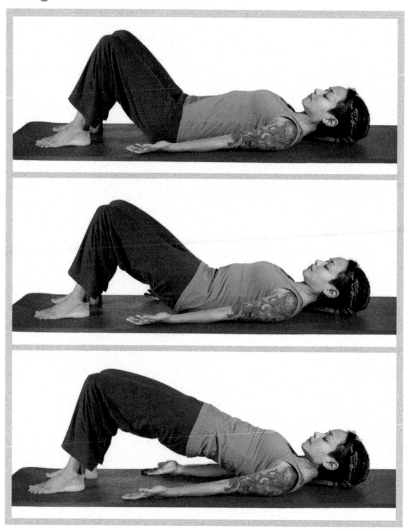

EXERCISE

Lie supine, with knees bent and hip width apart. Feet are aligned with the knees; heels 2–3 inches (5–8 cm) away from the sitting bones. Pelvis and spine are in a neutral position.

Inhale from top of head to tailbone, keeping pelvic floor relaxed *while* chin is down toward chest, to lengthen spine toward head to heavens.

- Exhale; pull pelvic floor toward the navel, posteriorly tilting hips. Imprint spine as the body lifts off the floor vertebrae by vertebrae until reaching scapulae, opening that back of heart to head.

- Activate legs, pressing feet firmly on the floor and engaging hamstrings and glutes.

- Inhale to create a diagonal line reaching from shoulders to knees, opening all gateways in the front of the body.

- Exhale; soften shoulders, chest, ribs, lumbars, and, last, tailbone, back to starting position, thus opening all gateways on the back of the body. Repeat.

IMAGERY

- Peel your spine off the floor, like a sticker, from tail to shoulder blades.

- At the top, imagine fireworks shooting from your shoulders through your knees.

- Lower your spine down like a fragile necklace, one crystal at a time.

AVOID

- hyperextending thoracic spine while hips are up.

- lowering spine down to the floor like a stiff plank. Find flexibility.

GATEWAYS

Begin with ground to groin, groin to gut, and gut to heart gateways while the head center reaches longer at the top of the head. Reverse the move from heart to gut to groin to ground.

NOAH'S EXTRA

This work is quite similar to Ida Rolf's pelvic lift which ended nearly every session she performed. As one research project showed years ago, the pelvic lift contributed to vagal tone. Doesn't it make sense that this simple work can help reset the vagus nerve?

Prone Pelvic Rock

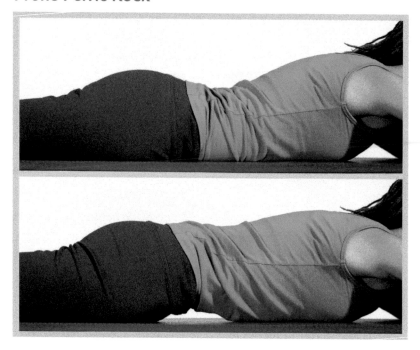

EXERCISE

Body relaxed, lie prone on the floor. Hands underneath forehead. Legs long and hip width apart.

- Inhale; initiate from groin center while reaching tailbone long. Lightly imprint belly to the floor; pelvis moves in an anterior tilt.

- Allow pelvic floor to be relaxed.

- Exhale; softly place tail on the floor, allowing belly to lift *while* pelvis moves into a posterior tilt.

- Lightly pull pelvic floor toward navel.

- Inhale to release into anterior tilt; exhale; repeat.

IMAGERY

- Visualize hot coal under the belly. Try to avoid it!

- Imagine your tail growing long and heavy as it reaches down toward and in between your feet.

AVOID

- tensing the upper torso.

- gripping the glutes.

GATEWAYS

Seemingly a simple exercise, Prone Pelvic Rock begins just a little beyond the groin center, where the tailbone leads the movement, waking up both the front and the back of the groin to gut and gut center. Meanwhile, gut to heart to heart center work as stabilizers. Ground to groin and heart to head to heavens create a subtle reach away from each other.

NOAH'S EXTRA

One of Liz's creations that needs little comment—only the awareness that the slower we go, the deeper we will find in our restrictions.

Swimming

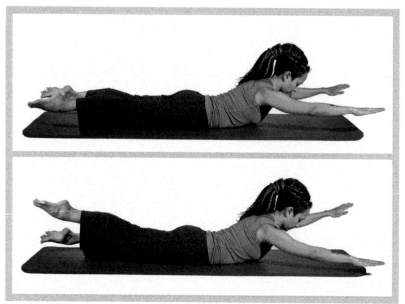

EXERCISE

Lie prone, with arms extended overhead, shoulder width apart.

- Open gut to heart: Extend arms overhead in line with your ears *while* legs extend, hip width apart.

- Head, arms, and legs hover an inch off the floor.

- Inhale; stretch the body long.

- Exhale; reach and raise opposite arm and opposite leg simultaneously.

- Inhale to return to position.

- Exhale; repeat on the other side.

- Stabilize groin to gut by lightly pulling navel toward the spine.

- Focus on the diagonal line that begins at navel and extends into opposite fingers and toes as you swim.

- Simultaneously emphasize lengthening and reaching from the top of head toward tailbone as well.

IMAGERY

- Visualize the body reaching to touch the front and back of the room with an oppositional energy orginating from the navel, reaching through and into the alternate fingertips and toes, the crown of your head growing taller toward to the front, while the tail grows longer from the back.

- With every inhale, grow longer throughout the whole body. With every exhale, rest in your new length.

AVOID

- sliding shoulders up to ears.

- allowing belly to drop, which hyperextends lower back.

GATEWAYS

As you alternate arms and legs, initiate the lengthening from the groin center that reaches down toward the groin to ground gateway to the toes, *while* groin to gut to head center, and gut to heart center, are pulled through the fingertips.

NOAH'S EXTRA

Explore putting more energy in individual fingers and toes to lengthen more: Move from the inner cuticle of the first finger and the outer cuticle of the big toe as you stretch with every breath.

Cat and Cow

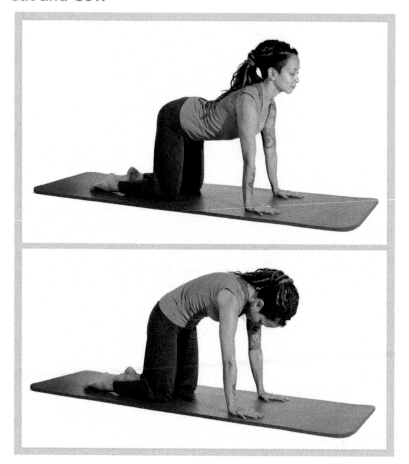

EXERCISE

On hands and knees, with torso facing down parallel to the floor, hands aligned with shoulders, and knees aligned with hips. Neutral spine from tailbone to top of head; elbows soft with inside of elbows facing each other.

- Inhale; allow ground to groin to relax and open.

- Exhale to curl tailbone under, like Tailbone Curl and Release on All Fours (pages 148–150), and continue to curl and push until spine is round, thus opening the back of all gateways.

- Inhale to reverse the movement; release pelvic floor, uncurling away from head center to elongate spine. Gaze slightly up to open heart to head.

- Emphasize rounding shoulders *back* to open heart center.

Sway Tail

- Reach your tailbone toward one side of your ribs and head. Repeat on the other side.

Tail Circles

- Combine Tailbone Curl and Release on All Fours (pages 148–150) and Sway Tail to draw circles with your tailbone.

- Add upper torso into movement to create a whole body exercise.

IMAGERY

- Cat and Cow—curl and round your back like an elephant with a long, heavy tail, then open chest as if to show off a beautiful necklace.

- Sway Tail—imagine you are able to sway your long tail from side to side toward your nose.

- Tail Circles—draw a circle with your tail in one direction; then draw a circle with your heart. Now try drawing both circles together one way; then explore drawing circles with them in opposite directions.

AVOID

- hyperextending the elbows.

- dropping the belly and/or hyperextending the lumbars.

GATEWAYS

Play with focusing on each center at a time, from ground to pelvic floor, to groin, to gut, to heart to head center. Then reverse the move from head to heart to gut to groin to ground.

NOAH'S EXTRA

Since my spine isn't supposed to move much (fused from T10 to L3, rods installed and removed years ago) this is a good one, but hard for me...as well as many people with back issues!

Sun Mermaid

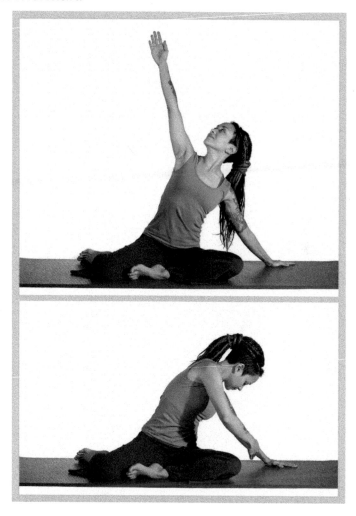

EXERCISE

Seated upright on the floor, prop sitting bones on pillow or blanket if necessary. Legs in Z-position or cross-legged.

- Inhale; elongate the spine from groin center to head to heavens, eyes looking forward.

- Float right arm toward the ceiling while left arm lengthens toward the floor.

- Exhale; right arm continues to reach up and toward left side of the body.

- Inhale into heart center while eyes gaze at right fingertips.

- Exhale; lower right arm down and under left side of the upper torso, opening back of heart center.

- Thorax curls and rotates as right arm arrives in between left arm and left side of the ribs. Gaze follows hand.

- Inhale; lift and return right arm up toward the ceiling. Exhale and repeat.

- Focus on the line from hand on the floor, across sternum, and through and toward raised arm.

- Maintain stable pelvis and legs as torso lifts up and over to the side.

IMAGERY

- Draw half a rainbow with the arm, fanning ribs as the body curls to the side. Then draw half a circle forward and under to opposite hand on the floor.

- Imagine that legs and hips are rooted deep into the earth, while spine sprouts from the ground and arms bloom.

AVOID

- hiking shoulder of arm on the floor up into ears.

- collapsing in torso.

GATEWAYS

Lift from the groin center to gut, tilting to the side through the gut center, to the heart. The heart center opens and travels through the arm rising up. Gazing at the fingertips, create a line from heart to head center to heavens.

NOAH'S EXTRA

I call this position the "Z" after Emmett Hutchins and Peter Melchior's Advanced Rolfing second-hour session. I hadn't thought to move the arms in this direction! Again, can you remember to keep sitting bones as equal into the floor as possible? Hint: It's impossible, but a worthy goal.

Spinal Twist with Open Chest

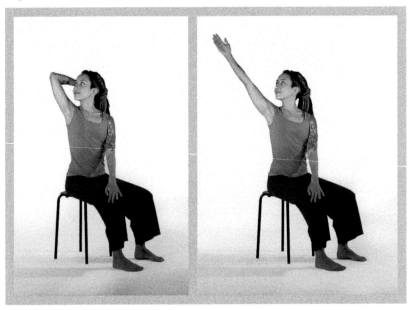

EXERCISE

Seated upright on a chair, legs parallel to the floor, knees at 90 degrees, and feet grounded on the floor.

- In starting position, raise right arm toward the sky.

- Bend elbow, placing right hand on the back of head, opening gut to heart, to heart center.

- Inhale; lightly press hand to head and head to hand to elongate spine toward head to heavens.

- Exhale; rotate upper torso to right from gut center while shoulders remain rested.

- Inhale to lengthen spine.

- Exhale to deepen the twist, maintaining your gaze at tip of the elbow.

Spinal Twist with Extending Arm

- As spine twists to the right, extend right arm while gaze follows right fingertips as arm reaches back.

- Inhale; create length from sternum to fingertips.

- Lower torso and legs remain firm and stable.

- Exhale; pull right ribs to return to center as right arm lowers. Repeat on other side.

IMAGERY

- Imagine there are three points connected from one side of the hip to the opposite elbow/hand and top of the head. As you twist, you are spiraling around, up and back.

- Visualize a whirlwind from tailbone traveling all the way up your spine and out of your lifted arm/elbow and head.

AVOID

- hiking shoulders.

- leaning the upper torso forward.

GATEWAYS

The spiraling movement begins at the groin center, grows through and toward the gut center and twists at the gut to heart gateway. The heart center opens as the elbow or extending arm reaches up, around and back. The following gaze triggers the heart to head gateway opening.

NOAH'S EXTRA

Isn't it interesting to think how both the office work population and nursing home residents could benefit from pulling their hands out of their hearts and gates above and below more frequently? For fun, change finger and hand positions and directions and observe the subtle differences.

Outer Orbit Channeling (*Wu Chi*) stance

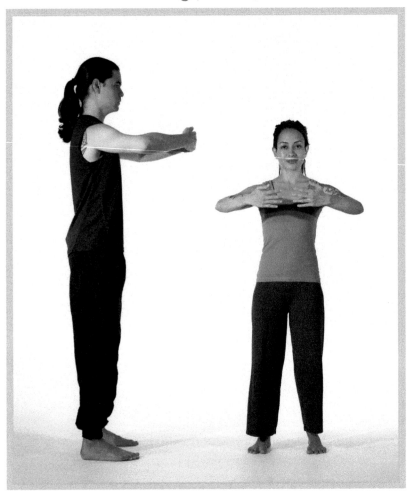

EXERCISE

Wu Chi stance is simple, yet powerful. Stand with feet shoulder
length apart. Point both feet parallel and forward, knees in line
with second toes. A slight external rotation may help in aligning the
knees to Bubbling Spring. Knees unlocked or gently bent, giving
the psoas a chance to release/relax into position. Stand tall from
feet to head. Back of the waist back, back of the neck back, and chin
slightly down to elongate the whole spine. Coccyx is untucked but
aimed downward to the ground.

- Inhale into soles of the feet.

- Exhale, working from ground to groin (or more like groin to ground), and allow your spine to elongate from the Bubbling Spring of your feet to the top of head while shoulders, arms, and fingers lengthen toward the ground.

- Float arms up at heart center. Form a circle with your arms as if you are holding a big ball. Fingers slightly open and pointing at each other.

- Upper torso—shoulders, elbows, and wrists—are relaxed as if floating in water. Breathe softly into navel.

- Keep spine and shoulders straight and aligned.

- Point of balance should be at the center top part of your feet.

IMAGERY

- As you inhale, visualize yourself reaching through and past the soles of your feet as your energy enters the ground. Feel the resistance of the earth as you reach deeper down into the earth.

- As you exhale, imagine you are on a trampoline. Release the resistance felt from the trampoline and allow the soft momentum response of the trampoline to lift and ripple up through your spine. At the same time, visualize an invisible line that pulls you toward the heavens.

AVOID

- lifting the chin up and away from the chest.

- over-tucking the tailbone, or pushing the pelvis toward the front.

- slouching or tensing the shoulders.

- stiffening and tensing the chest.

- shifting body weight toward the heels.

GATEWAYS

Maintain emphasis on ground to groin gateway that roots deep in the ground while still reaching each and every gateway toward head to heavens. Imagine this line spreading into the arms and fingertips, creating a warm circular energy around the heart center.

NOAH'S EXTRA

This is a more traditional tai chi-like stance and introduction to energy work. If it doesn't resonate for you, pass it by. If it does, you can spend the next 20 years exploring it! I'd also encourage us all to spend more time grounding our inner arches into the floor on this and other standing postures... Can you settle, safely, into your feet?

Standing Rolldown

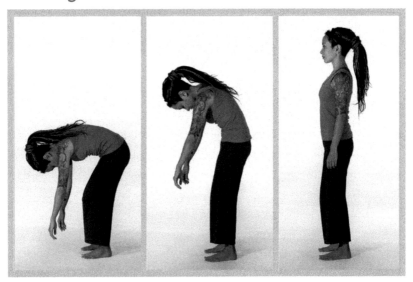

EXERCISE

- Begin in standing *Wu Chi* position (see page 228).

- Inhale; nod chin to lengthen the back of neck.

- Exhale; roll and round spine forward and down, opening all gateways from head center to groin center toward the floor.

- Arms, shoulders, and head are heavy and relaxed.

- Pelvic floor gently pulled toward navel; back of waist back.

- Pause to inhale and exhale, and continue.

- Knees bend slightly as hands reach the floor.

- Inhale at the bottom of the movement, releasing and relaxing navel and pelvic floor.

- Exhale; lightly pull pelvic floor and navel as spine rolls up back to starting position. Repeat.

IMAGERY

- Peel your body off a wall slowly.

- Imagine you are a candle melting to the floor.

AVOID

- locking or hyperextending the knees.

- lowering the body as a whole, like one big plank, instead of articulating the spine.

- stiffening the shoulders and arms.

GATEWAYS

As the spine rolls forward and toward the floor, the front of the body, specifically the abdominals, will contract; thus the back muscles of the body will release and stretch. As the spine rolls back up to standing, the back muscles contract, allowing the front body to release and open.

Understanding that the gateways stem from both the front and back side of the body, begin in reverse from the heavens to head center, curling the spine and opening the back of all the gateways toward the pelvic floor to ground.

For me, this hearkens to my forward bend against a wall. Slide the head down a wall, *while* pulling the low back up, *while* grounding in the pigeon-toed stance *with* grounded inner arches. This stretch truly calls on most centers and gateways. I'm going to issue a challenge to us all: You'll be happier if/when you can get your palms to actually touch the floor in front of you as you bend forward. Remember, this is a challenge, not a command! Perhaps you'll need to stand in front of a step, or two, and put your palms there. Explore.

Sky Hands

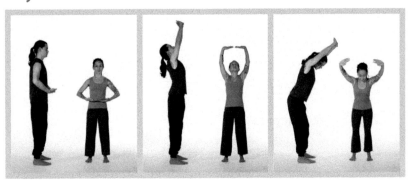

EXERCISE

In *Wu Chi* stance (page 228). Both hands at navel level, with fingertips facing each other and palms facing up. Knees hip width apart.

- Inhale; bend elbows and raise both palms together. At chest level rotate both palms outward to face up above head.

- Exhale; extend arms and stretch the entire line of body from ground to heaven with a slight back bend. Chin up to gaze in between fingers.

- Inhale; hinge forward from hips, maintaining a straight spine.

- Exhale; keeping palms up, allow head to drop in between stretched arms to elongate the whole torso.

- Return to starting position and allow palms to slowly float down toward belly and sides of body.

IMAGERY

- Visualize carrying clouds gently from below to above your head. Give the clouds an extra nudge to push them back to the sky where they belong.

AVOID

- hyperextending the back.

- hyperexending the elbows and knees.

- lifting shoulders toward the ears.

GATEWAYS

A beautiful stretch from deep within the soles of the feet, ground through to heavens with the movement initiating from the groin to gut and emphasizing the heart center, up/out and into the palms of the hands.

NOAH'S EXTRA

Do you see how this asks for my "Willow X"? Once you've achieved this posture, why not ask for more movement; slowly, deeply, with awareness.

Pluck the Flower

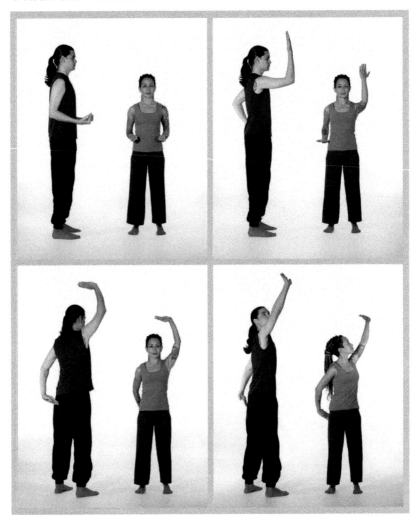

EXERCISE

In *Wu Chi* stance (page 228) with elbows bent and forearms parallel to the floor, at lower ribcage level.

- Inhale; lift one forearm at 90 degrees from your elbow with palm facing and aligned with your face. The alternate hand simultaneously pulls back, brushing the side of ribs, palm facing up.

- Rotate both palms.

- The arm with palm facing you will stretch upward and in front of torso, while both palms begin to face up toward the sky.

- The other arm by the side of ribs, with palm facing up, will rotate and move behind torso to face and press down toward the floor.

- Exhale; reach both palms apart up/down respectively, opening gut to heart center. Keep arms stretched without locking elbows.

- Inhale; twist from groin to gut toward the side of upper arm (i.e., if right arm is up, twist to right side).

- Look up through fingers of upper hand to open heart to head.

- Exhale; continue to press into both palms more from front and back of torso, stretching deeper along your arms.

- Float both palms in a circular motion to return to starting position.

- Pelvis and shoulders remain aligned.

- Reach and stretch arms away from the gut center.

IMAGERY

- Visualize pushing against the ground and the ceiling at the same time.

- Imagine an invisible line from the upper palm connected to the top of the head. As you push up, your palm is pulling your head as well as the entire torso up to straighten and lengthen the spine further.

AVOID

- tensing and locking arms and hands.

- locking knees.

- tensing shoulders.

REPETITION

- Traditionally three times on each side.

GATEWAYS

As in *Wu Chi* stance, the ground to groin roots downward to stabilize the movement while still subtly extending up and through to head to heavens. Groin to gut open when rotating hips to the side. The gut to heart shines into the heart center through and into both palms, as the hands push groin to ground and head to heavens from the center.

NOAH'S EXTRA

Explore: Allow your elbows to be in charge of upper body movements; then wrists, then fingers, and even experiment with thinking all movement comes from the shoulders.

Heaven and Earth

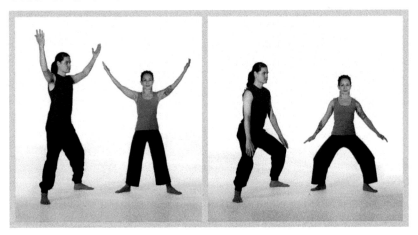

EXERCISE

Feet are double shoulder width apart. Externally rotate both legs out at a 45 degree angle; knees straight with slight bend. Maintain knees aligned with Bubbling Spring. Pelvis is relaxed, and back is straight.

- Inhale; float arms above and away from shoulder line.

- Exhale; lower arms and bend knees slowly and, at the same time, open groin to gut gateway and heart center simultaneously.

- Arms are soft and allow gravity to pull down shoulders, elbows, wrists, and fingers (following that order).

- Repeat, inhaling to straighten legs and float arms up.

- The muscles work more when the movement is slowed down.

- As knees bend, adductors stretch, and pelvis remains relaxed to allow spine to stay elongated while the entire body lowers to the ground.

IMAGERY

- Visualize there are clouds under your hands. As you inhale, imagine the clouds floating your hands up. Exhale; allow arms to float downward, caressing the clouds.

- When bending knees, feel that you are entering the ground from the perineum and feel the deepening stability from the pressure on the sides of your feet.

AVOID

- over-stretching arms too high and too far away from shoulder line, which can create rigidity in the movement.

- locking your knees when raising arms up. This can create a blockage and reduces fluidity in the movement.

GATEWAYS

Root from ground to groin, with legs open to free the groin center and groin to gut. The arms free the gut to heart and open the heart center. All the while, the line elongates the body equally from gut to ground, and from gut to heavens.

Again, tai chi at its best. What seems like a simple direction could consume years of practice! And remember, the slower you allow yourself to explore, the more new scenery you find.

Pull Open the Bow Pluck the Flower

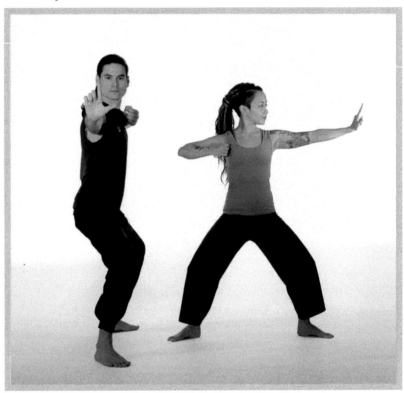

EXERCISE

Legs remain in Heaven and Earth stance (page 236).

- Inhale; float arms above and away from shoulder line. One hand forms an L with index finger and thumb.

- Extend arm in line with shoulders.

- The other hand forms a fist. Exhale; bend arm and pull fist toward chest.

- Eyes gaze to hand formed into the L.

- Knees remain bent in this exercise.

IMAGERY

- Hold a bow steady and pull the string of the bow with every inhale.

AVOID

- arching the spine and/or anteriorly tilting the pelvis.

- stiffening the chest.

- locking the arm.

GATEWAYS

Just as with Heaven and Earth, root from ground to groin, with legs open and stable to free the groin to gut. The play of flexing and extending each arm moves the heart center. The body elongates equally from the center of gut to ground, and from gut to heavens.

NOAH'S EXTRA

Here we're adding a bit of neck roll similar to what I've been suggesting. Can you remember the idea of neck rolls happening from any of the many spinal segments?

Appendix C

"Maturity"

If, as Ida Rolf is reputed to have said, "Maturity is the ability to discern finer and finer layers of distinction...," then this last, short appendix is a step to maturity for movement therapists. Here I challenge you to move forward with your new knowledge: past my writings, past the excellent awareness exercises and challenges Rob and Liz have presented, and further into the concept of training both self and clients to more fully observe and explore patterns, distortions, restrictions, and lack of movement in our/their own bodies.

So here you'll find that my directions get shorter, less specific, and more challenging. You've noticed my exercises haven't included photos—mostly because I believe each of us needs to find the individual bits that have become stuck. There is no "one size fits all!" Take your time, think about the words, explore, and you'll be rewarded.

I often use the word "while," which takes on a special significance for me. I believe we need to get better and better at incorporating more directions into our rubber band; therefore, whenever I ask for a movement, l try to find that second, third, and fourth stretch. For me, "while" means: look/feel around and find another way to softly and safely challenge yourself. Then add yet another movement that might just bring feelings to be processed and released as well as physical release.

Stretching Any from All

Remember the "Willow X" concept from Appendix A and mentioned briefly in B? Explore moving your body in all planes and directions. First, plant your feet—flattened into the ground, shoulder width or wider. Raise the arms so as to form an X; next stretch in any direction you can find. Push/pull the genitals downforward *while* the waist moves upback. Focus next on mild twisting...you may need to stop and explore here for a good while, to find low and mid back tensions. Any and every center can and will be stretched from all other centers and gateways with a bit of experimentation. To get even more sophisticated, explore drawing horizontal circles with the belly button and mid body *while* you stay grounded in your inner arches. Then focus on allowing the hips to go clockwise and counterclockwise. Next, put any and all of these stretches together!

To get even more complicated: *While* you're twisting, flexing, and stretching above, what happens if you find a vertebra several bones higher than your primary fulcrum, then decide to *both lift and laterally flex* from that spot as you work on the lower fulcrum?

In the above stretch we could also use elbows as the fulcrum from which we tugged... What if the Willow X uses the proximal joints of elbows and knees instead of the distal hands and feet areas? Pretty much any experiment you want to explore is asking yet another part of the body to wake up and move.

Grounding in the Outer Malleoli

Stand: ground feet anywhere from 12 to 30 inches (30–75 cm) apart and straight on (depending on what you want and plan to explore, feet may turn out sometimes). Find the lateral longitudinal arches of the feet (the length of the outside of foot) and explore asking that line to take weight; once you've found them, you realize a new line and stance. Can you put weight equally into both outer feet? Can you feel an interesting extra bit of stretch on the outer malleoli? Now, imagine you can shift weight into a diagonal line that goes from just behind the little toe, across to the big toe, but just in back of all toes. Can you see how this line both asks you to put weight in a new spot, but also activates your Bubbling Spring? With your weight spread equally, imagine your inner arches, and, in fact, everything on the plantar surface not yet touching the floor, can get longer and flatter, relaxing your arches while keeping weight in that line behind the toes. Settle, balance, feel, and breathe.

Next flex and settle your knees slightly; pull the groin/genitals downforward, then your back and belly button upback. Stay in knee flexion, then move on. Allow the back of the head to lift back upback and add this awareness with breath. Now, move *something*, slowly. Explore the body and on finding what complains; observe gently, compassionately, but directly, with breath.

Then explore a spinal forward-and-back undulation; imagine each vertebra on the chain can be the one to push furthest forward while a stuck space in your neck is being pulled away by a long and tall head.

After finding all these spots, return to the malleoli, especially the outer (though inner may speak louder to you). Try to find your lower tibia and fibula as they relate to the foot bones *while* you stay aware of everything above. By the way, do your knees complain when you find the ankles?

Cock the Hip

Standing, one leg is grounded straight and short; second foot and leg moves slightly out to side. Put the most weight in straight leg; then allow self to tighten hip joint and quadratus lumborum (QL). Tighten, breathe, release. Find and feel that QL, then exaggerate the tension you feel. Inhale, find it; exhale, release. Explore in any order of breath and awareness and movement that works for you.

After exploring the QL, allow yourself to find the other tight and weak spot(s) up and down the line (very possibly knees, but might be ankles, etc.).

Stress the Clavicle

Imagine that the clavicle, which is the only bony attachment of the arm to the skeleton, could be stretched, stressed, and exercised more fully. Find a sturdy counter, table, or railing that comes up to about the bottom of your sacrum. Face away; place your hands on the surface behind you and lift yourself with your arms, letting the wrists take the weight and stressing the sternoclavicular junction. Realize you're (a) opening shoulders, (b) hanging the spine from the shoulders instead of vice versa, and (c) able to lift your head and neck out of the stuck spots you're bound to find as you work to open this neglected aspect of your line.

Front Legs

If we allow ourselves to practice four-legged animal walks, we'll find our front legs don't take much weight. Explore allowing more weight into the heels of the front feet (hands); try walking with more weight in the toes of the front legs. Explore twisting and flexing while you're exploring the use of front legs.

Conclusions

Simply put, I'm most interested in getting clients, and self, to learn to move any of the four centers as far away from the rest as possible:

- Groin away from gut, heart, and head, or any two or three.

- Gut away from groin, heart, and head, or any two or three.

- Heart away from head, gut, and groin, or any two or three.

- Head away from heart, gut, and groin, or any two or three.

Most mature: I practice walking, standing, and sitting with my waist back and heart upfront, on purpose. When I ground feet in Bubbling Spring on that diagonal line just behind the toes, lightly flex my knees, bring genitals downforward, waist upback, heart upfront, and head upback, I feel I'm on my line and on my purpose.

Stop and wait for the message of your work! This is what we don't do, too much of the time. In life as well as in bodymindcore explorations, we move quickly, in achievement mode instead of exploration mode. Allow your bodymindcore to talk to you, and remember that communication includes listening! The challenge is to take the step beyond simply joining gateways and centers in the stretches, to start really looking for symmetry, length, and openness; and for finding those bits you like to hide or try to ignore.

If maturity is as Ida Rolf describes, can we consciously reach for the next deepest layer daily? I hope this message resonates: move...stretch...breathe...go deeper, slower, more deeply, more slowly wherever you go. My most mature advice to you: Challenge yourself so you can challenge your clients. How do we move more deliberately, with more awareness, into more hidden areas, more of the time? This is bodymindcore.

I'm a believer that any person with a degree of patience can find and repair or heal many aches and pains they find in their body—if they look at, listen to, and challenge that body. We're all still works in progress—I haven't cured all my ills! But I have overcome many through attention and intention, and I celebrate where I am while I thank and forgive the past. And the deeper I'm going, the slower I travel.

Good luck in your bodymindcore journey, with clients and with yourself.

Notes

CHAPTER 1

1. CORE is an acronym for Center Of Right Energy; from personal class notes. Also see "Core Energetics," available at http://psychology.wikia.com/wiki/Core_Energetics, accessed on September 28, 2016.
2. Bond, Mary (2007) *The New Rules of Posture*. Rochester, VT: Healing Arts Press, p. 93.
3. Schultz, Louis and Feitis, Rosemary (1996) *The Endless Web*. Berkeley, CA: North Atlantic Books, p. 36.
4. Levine, Peter (2010) *In an Unspoken Voice*. Berkeley, CA: North Atlantic Books, p. 15.
5. Sarno, John (2006) *The Divided Mind*. New York, London, Toronto, Sydney: Harper, p. 20.
6. Radio interview/transcript of Stephen Porges, with Ruth Buzyinski (2014) "The Polyvagal Theory for Treating Trauma," available at http://stephenporges.com/index. php/component/content/article/5-popular-articles/25-nicabm-the-polyvagal-theory-for-treating-trauma, accessed on 23 January 2017; Porges, Stephen (2011) *The Polyvagal Theory: Neurophysiologial Foundations of Emotions, Attachment, Communication, and Self-Regulation*. New York: W. W. Norton.
7. Bergland, Christopher (2016) "Vagus Nerve Stimulation Dramatically Reduces Inflammation." *Psychology Today*, July 6. Available at https://www.psychologytoday. com/blog/the-athletes-way/201607/vagus-nerve-stimulation-dramatically-reduces-inflammation, accessed on September 28, 2016.
8. Chaitow, Leon, in Bond, *The New Rules of Posture*, p. ix.

CHAPTER 2

1. Feitis, Rosemary and Rolf, Ida P. (1978) *(Ida Rolf Talks about) Rolfing and Physical Reality*. New York, Haegerstown, San Francisco, London: Harper and Row, p. 26.
2. Quoted in Feitis and Rolf, *(Ida Rolf Talks about) Rolfing and Physical Reality*, p. 26.

3. Noah Karrasch's student notes, Rolf Institute, 1986.
4. Schultz, Louis and Feitis, Rosemary (1996) *The Endless Web*. Berkeley, CA: North Atlantic Books, p. 49.
5. Egoscue, Pete (2011) *Pain Free Living*. New York: Ethos, p. 2.
6. Nelson, Douglas (2013) *The Mystery of Pain*. London and Philadelphia: Singing Dragon, p. 15.
7. Nelson, *The Mystery of Pain*, p. 14.
8. Egoscue, *Pain Free Living*, p. 2.
9. Levine, Peter (2015) *Trauma and Memory*. Berkeley, CA: North Atlantic Books, pp. 48–50.
10. Wall, Patrick, in Nelson, *The Mystery of Pain*, p. 125.

CHAPTER 3

1. Frank, Jerome and Frank, Julia (1961, 1991) *Persuasion and Healing*. Baltimore, MD and London: Johns Hopkins University Press, pp. 40–3.
2. Distilling pp. 40–3 of Frank and Frank, *Persuasion and Healing*.
3. Levine, *Trauma and Memory*, pp.62-3.
4. Bond, Mary (2007) *The New Rules of Posture*. Rochester, VT: Healing Arts Press, p. 199.
5. Karrasch, Noah (2015) *Getting Better at Getting People Better*. London and Philadelphia: Singing Dragon.

CHAPTER 4

1. Shaffer, Fred, McCraty, Rollin, and Zerr, Christopher (2014) "A Heart Is Not a Metronome: An Integrative Review of the Heart's Anatomy and Heart Rate Variability." *Frontiers in Psychology*, 5, 1040. Available at www.ncbi.nlm.nih.gov/pmc/articles/PMC4179748, accessed on September 29, 2016.
2. Bergland, Christopher (2016) "Vagus Nerve Stimulation Dramatically Reduces Inflammation." *Psychology Today*, July 6. Available at https://www.psychologytoday.com/blog/the-athletes-way/201607/vagus-nerve-stimulation-dramatically-reduces-inflammation, accessed on September 28, 2016.
3. Schultz, Louis and Feitis, Rosemary (1996) *The Endless Web*. Berkeley, CA: North Atlantic Books, p. 47.

CHAPTER 5

1. Egoscue, Pete (2011) *Pain Free Living*. New York: Ethos, p. 25.
2. Gladwell, Malcolm (2005) *Blink*. New York: Back Bay Books/Little, Brown and Co, pp. 124–5.

CHAPTER 6

1. Schultz, Louis and Feitis, Rosemary (1996) *The Endless Web*. Berkeley, CA: North Atlantic Books, p. 83.
2. Bond, Mary (2007) *The New Rules of Posture*. Rochester, VT: Healing Arts Press, p. 4.
3. Myers, Thomas (2009) *Anatomy Trains: Myofascial Meridians for Manual and Movement Therapists*. Edinburgh: Churchill Livingstone/Elsevier.
4. Levine, Peter (2015) *Trauma and Memory*. Berkeley, CA: North Atlantic Books, pp. 145–6.
5. Schultz and Feitis, *The Endless Web*, p. 109.
6. Bond, *The New Rules of Posture*, p. 4.

CHAPTER 8

1. Karrasch, Noah (2012) *Freeing Emotions and Energy (Through Myofascial Release).* London and Philadelphia: Singing Dragon; (2015) *Getting Better at Getting People Better.* London and Philadelphia: Singing Dragon.
2. Bond, Mary (2007) *The New Rules of Posture.* Rochester, VT: Healing Arts Press.
3. Cantwell, Alan (2004) "Dr. Wilhelm Reich: Scientific Genius – or Medical Madman?," *New Dawn*, 84, available at http://newdawnmagazine.com/Article/Dr_Wilhelm_ Reich_Scientific_Genius.html (accessed on October 27, 2016)—a great article that talks about Reich in depth!
4. Schultz, Louis and Feitis, Rosemary (1996) *The Endless Web.* Berkeley, CA: North Atlantic Books, p. 35.

Index

slow and low breaths 110, 128–9, 142–5,
152–5
social communication and engagement
system 25
solar plexus
chakra 94, 96, 106–8
opening exercise 172–4
Somatic Experiencing (SE) 22, 46, 56–7
Somersaulting Turtle 169
sphenoid bones 97, 118–19
spinal curves 94, 120
Spinal Twist with Extending Arm 227
Spinal Twist with Open Chest 226
stance 99
Standing Rolldown 230–2
starfish analogy 17–18, 63–4
strength 82, 84
Stress the Clavicle 246
Stretch/Awareness exercises
bandhas 210
contracting and relaxing 210–11
creating 207
gateways 208–9
incorporating multiple centers 212–39
movement modalities used 209–10
rules for 208
teaching to explore 211
teaching to stretch from all areas 211
stretching
with breath 71
maximizing effect of 71–2, 83
movement and posture 73–6
personal lines 72–3, 80
points of star 19, 28
rubber band analogy 71–2, 207–8
straps 88, 160
Stretching Any from All 244
suboccipital muscles 96, 119, 198–202
Sun Mermaid 223–5
survival chakra 94, 96
Swimming 219–20
sympathetic nervous system (SNS) 25–6, 48,
55–6, 58–9
symptoms 67–8

tactile skills 43–5, 50, 73
Tailbone Curl and Release on All Fours
148–50
tails
of body star 98, 101, 103
wagging 101, 103, 139–40, 210–11
Tapping Toes 136–7
"texter's neck" 78, 97
therapy
and breath 53–4, 61

coaxing skills 48–51
communication skills 41–3
hard and soft 49–50
layers of 45–6
persuasion and healing 44–6
tactile skills 43–5
for traumatic memories 46–8
see also client participation
third eye/head chakra 94, 96, 116–18
throat
chakra 94, 96, 113–16, 184–5
opening 116, 122, 185
tibialis posterior muscle 32, 100, 134–6
tightening/tension
muscles 21–2, 28
our cores 32–3, 39
and self-esteem 110
and strength 82
worsening pain 31, 48
"titration" 46
tonic immobility 22–3, 28
tools *see* exercise equipment
touch 43–5, 50, 73
trauma
body responses to 21–3, 28
breath to "shake out" 38, 60–1
and fibromyalgia 58–9
memories of
and brain 36–7
renegotiating 46–7
and nervous system 25–6
"trauma response" mode 36–7
Turtle 168–9

upper erector muscles 96, 116–18
Upper Star (GV23) 18, 64

"vagal brake" 26, 56
"vagal pacemakers" 55
"vagal reset" 55–6, 61, 110, 118
vagal system 25, 57, 59
vagal tone 56, 217
vagus nerve 23–5, 55–6, 58, 118, 217
ventral vagus nerve 25, 58

walking 87, 99–100, 131–2, 246–7
Wall, P. 39, 43, 59
Welcoming Arms, Hug Yourself 182–4
words
giving thought to 90, 243
inviting self-exploration 44
safe 43
use of 89–90

Zerr, C. 54